SELF-AWARENESS IN HEALTH CARE

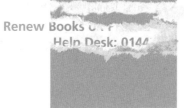

Also by Dev M. Rungapadiachy

INTERPERSONAL COMMUNICATION AND PSYCHOLOGY FOR HEALTH CARE
PROFESSIONALS: Theory and practice

Self-Awareness in Health Care

Engaging in Helping Relationships

Dev M. Rungapadiachy

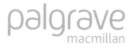

First published 2008 by
PALGRAVE MACMILLAN
Houndmills, Basingstoke, Hampshire RG21 6XS and
175 Fifth Avenue, New York, N.Y. 10010
Companies and representatives throughout the world

PALGRAVE MACMILLAN is the global academic imprint of the Palgrave Macmillan division of St. Martin's Press, LLC and of Palgrave Macmillan Ltd. Macmillan® is a registered trademark in the United States, United Kingdom and other countries. Palgrave is a registered trademark in the European Union and other countries.

ISBN-13: 978–0–230–01988–1 paperback
ISBN-10: 0–230–01988–9 paperback

Learning Resources
Centre

13115464

This book is printed on paper suitable for recycling and made from fully managed and sustained forest sources. Logging, pulping and manufacturing processes are expected to conform to the environmental regulations of the country of origin.

A catalogue record for this book is available from the British Library.

10   9   8   7   6   5   4   3   2   1
17 16 15 14 13 12 11 10 09 08

Printed and bound in China

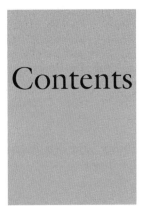

Contents

List of Figures

List of Tables

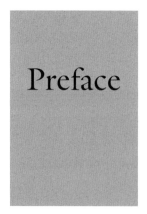

Preface

It is often said that academic books are written in order to reflect emerging themes of the era during which they were written. *Self-Awareness in Health Care* does not contradict this trend as it has made an attempt to address a contemporary notion of the nature and process of health care delivery. One of the buzzwords in health care is engagement, the danger, however, is that it runs the risk of remaining nothing but a catchphrase unless one is prepared to examine its meanings. Truly engaging patients in their own care is not as simple as it sounds because of two principal barriers, namely, practitioners and patients themselves. For example, engagement can only take place if I, as a practitioner, believe in its potential benefit to patients, thus actively working towards facilitating that process. Moreover, I can achieve this if and *only if* patients are willing participants. This suggests that a patient-centered approach would best suit both practitioners and patients. Central to patient-centered care is the skill of empathy where practitioners attempt to understand the experience of illness and discomfort from patients' perspectives. Literature on empathy suggests two schools of thought: those who believe that it only exists as a theoretical concept and that translating empathy to practice is beyond human capacity, and those who are more optimistic about empathy as a means to connect with patients. My personal orientation favours the second school of thought; however, when I read in students' essays that none of them have problems empathising with their patients I began to wonder exactly how they demonstrate this empathy. Here lies the problem: very few are able to explain the process; however, most give the impression that empathy is something that they carry in their pockets to distribute at will to their patients, *with a smile on my face I empathise with my patients.* It is almost comical, but at the same time seriously worrying how the notion of empathy is conceptualised. My sentiment is that the actual display of empathy on the part of practitioners is secondary to patients' perceived empathy. When patients are able to feel that I have made a genuine attempt at understanding their situation then perhaps I am on the right path towards developing empathic understanding.

Whilst no step-by-step guide is offered in *Self-Awareness in Health Care*, the very essence of translating empathy into practice rests with practitioners' ability to listen attentively. Crucial to listening skills is the notion of self-awareness. Perhaps, it would not be an exaggeration to state that, generally, people have a tendency to shy away from the topic of self-awareness. Admittedly, the journey to self-discovery can be uncomfortable and painful at times. However, the reward outweighs this sense of discomfort and pain because as a health care professional one becomes a much more efficient practitioner by engaging patients in their own care. *Self-Awareness in Health Care* emphasises the need to involve individuals in their own care, thus moving a step closer to addressing the imbalance of power that exists between patients and health care professionals.

Dev M. Rungapadiachy

Acknowledgements

Writing *Self-Awareness in Health Care* was meant to be a collaborative venture between myself and my two colleagues Jack Morris and Steve Howarth. Unfortunately, due to our personal and professional schedules and my desperate need for control, this book has become a personal project. Jack and Steve, in taking full authorship of *Self-Awareness in Health Care*, I recognise and acknowledge your contributions and thank you both for your help and advice throughout that process. My sincere thanks to Lynda Thompson who believed in me and Sarah Lodge for keeping me informed. A special thank you to you Darren for your creative skills reflected in all the drawings in *Self-Awareness in Health Care*. Last, but not least, to my wife Devi for patiently enduring the 'lows' and in particular, those of the last two years of my life. Devi, none of what I have been able to achieve academically would have been possible without you by my side.

Notes on Contributors

Steve Howarth is Senior Nursing Lecturer and Programme Manager for Mental Health, University of Leeds.

Jack Morris is Lecturer in Mental Health, University of Leeds.

Dev M. Rungapadiachy is Lecturer in Psychology and Mental Health, University of Leeds.

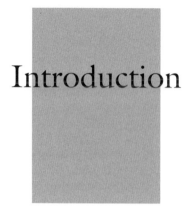

Introduction

The principal emphasis of *Self-Awareness in Health Care* stems from the idea that individuals arguably, through not fault of their own, are disempowered by virtue of taking on the role of patients. It would be fair to say that the patient role has a tendency to inhibit the range of activities individuals are able to engage in, either because they are physically or psychologically unable to do so or because of the constraints imposed by the health care environment, or both. Thus, it could be argued that illness per se can be seen as a stressful experience as in some cases individuals lose their sense of control and may have to rely on health care professionals in order to regain some normality in their lives. Here lies the crucial factor: that health care professionals heavily influence patients' experience of health services. As health care professionals, we may say that we care for our patients; however, observed non-verbal behaviour may contradict our notion of caring. Practitioners' self-awareness therefore becomes a prerequisite for engaging with patients as well as engaging them in their own care. Health care professionals need to be sufficiently transparent in order to gain the patients' trust that is considered to be essential for the development of therapeutic relationships. With this in mind, *Self-Awareness in Health Care* is structured in three parts, where each part relates to a particular theme; (1) On Developing Self-Awareness: A Way of Engaging (2) Self-Awareness and The Person's Experience, and (3) Communication, Engagement, and the Helping Relationship. The theme of self-awareness is maintained throughout the book and in some instances this is attempted through a series of exercises that encourage the reader to translate theoretical concepts into practice. Some of the exercises require a cautious approach in view of their content, while others encourage self-disclosure that may in itself cause personal discomfort. The main principle that underpins these exercises is that by sensing and feeling the experience, practitioners should in theory be more skilled at demonstrating empathic understanding towards patients.

Chapter 1 offers a theoretical understanding of self-awareness in an attempt to demonstrate how it can be a valuable skill in enhancing one's own efficiency as a health care professional. There is an argument to suggest that individuals possess a wealth of self-knowledge based on their past experience. However, much of this information is believed to be outside the realm of conscious awareness, hence justifying the need to understand the implication lack of self-awareness can have on the health care professional–patient relationship. Self-awareness and the person's experience of illness are addressed in Chapters 2, 3, 4, and 5, where factors such as stress and vulnerability, power and empowerment, emotion of loss, and anger and aggression are explored respectively. The starting point of communication, engagement, and the helping relationship is with Chapter 6, which addresses language as a forerunner to human communication. Chapter 7 discusses the notion of intrapersonal communication, where values, beliefs, and attitudes are found to be significant elements in human interaction. Interpersonal communication and interpersonal skills are the topics of Chapter 8, where inclusion, control, and affection are identified as three of people's interpersonal needs, thus necessitating interpretive, goal, role, self, and message competencies. Finally, Chapter 9 attempts to situate the notion of engagement in practice through a structured model of care.

PART I

On Developing Self-Awareness

A Way of Engaging

Engagement is one of the buzzwords of the twenty-first century and one could even go so far as to say that it is hailed as the essence of care. The word engagement is taken to mean *involving people in their own care*, to *encourage them to take an active part in what happens to them when they become ill*, to *collaborate in their care*, to *work in partnership with health care professionals*. According to Kravitz and Melnikow (2001), political trends, thinking on ethics, and research on health services have contributed to the belief that patients ought to be more involved in their own care. Moreover, evidence seems to suggest that engaging patients in their own care may be an important influence on health outcomes (Kaplan, Greenfield, & Ware, 1989). However, from a practical perspective, engaging patients in their own care can be a complex undertaking, and changes are needed on the part of health care practitioners in order to 'move policy from lip service to a reality' (Thomson, Bowling, & Moss, 2001, p. i1). Every health care professional would like to feel that the care they offer is guided by the health care needs of their patients. There are instances where this is not always the case. Perhaps, it would be much more accurate to state that approaches to care delivery are dictated by institutional and professional obstacles (Rungapadiachy, 2003). For example, Kennelly and Bowling (2001) argue that clinical judgement is influenced by socio-demographic characteristics of the patient, stereotyping, and health care resources. A further crucial factor that can significantly influence treatment and care is practitioners' personal beliefs, values, and attitudes. Rakow (2007) argues that if two doctors differ in their beliefs about the relative merits of different treatments, then one would expect each doctor to have his or her own individual preference. Given that both are doctors it follows that they will be on equal par to express their rationale for choice. However, the dynamic will most likely be different if one party is subordinate to the other by virtue of role definition. Patients in general tend to show a deferential attitude towards practitioners during the practitioner–patient relationship unless of course practitioners try to readdress the imbalance of power between the two parties. One way this could be achieved is through what Rogers (1967) called *empathic understanding*, described as a form of emotional knowing of another person's experiencing and feeling (see Chapters 1 and 9). It could be argued that the starting point to understanding a patient's feeling and experience rests with practitioners' awareness of their own experience and feeling. Moreover, self-awareness on the part of practitioners could be seen as crucial to the process of engaging patients in their own care. Part one addresses issues related to self-awareness.

References

Kaplan, S., Greenfield, S., and Ware, J. (1989). Assessing the effects of physician-patient interactions on the outcomes of chronic disease. *Medical Care*, 27(3) (supplement), S110–S127.

Kennelly, C. and Bowling, A. (2001). Suffering in deference: a focus group study of older cardiac patients' preferences for treatment and perceptions of risk. *Quality in Health Care*, 10 (supplement I), i23–i28.

Kravitz, R. L. and Melnikow, J. (2001). Engaging patients in medical decision-making. *British Medical Journal*, 323, 584–585.

Rakow, T. (2001). Differences in belief about likely outcomes account for differences in doctors' treatment preferences: but what accounts for the differences in belief? *Quality in Health Care*, 10 (supplement I), i44–i49.

Rogers, C. R. (1967). *On Becoming a Person: A Therapist's View of Psychotherapy*. London: Constable.

Rungapadiachy, D. M. (2003). *The Role of the Mental Health Nurse: A Comparison of the Perceptions of Mental Health Nurses, Pre-Post Registration, and Experienced Mental Health Nurses*. Unpublished Thesis. University of Leeds, Leeds.

Thomson, R., Bowling, A., and Moss, F. (2001). *Quality and Safety in Health Care*, 10 (supplement 1), i1.

1

Self-Awareness

Dev M. Rungapadiachy

After reading this chapter you should be able to

▦ Discuss the concept of self-awareness.

▦ Demonstrate how your self-awareness can help you understand others.

▦ Apply self-awareness to your practice.

Introduction

It could be argued that one of the characteristics that differentiate human from all other animals is our ability to think consciously in deliberate, complex, and abstract ways about ourselves (Leary & Buttermore, 2003). According to Vorauer and Ross (1999), individuals possess a wealth of self-knowledge based on their past behaviours and their inner thoughts, feelings, goals, and intentions. Moreover, much of this information is private and not readily available to others. One could add that some people may not even recognise their inner thoughts and feelings unless of course they make a conscious attempt to do so. Even then these may be too traumatic to assimilate into their system (this point will become clear as the chapter develops). The question Vorauer and Ross (1999, p. 416) posed is, "do people realize the extent to which their self-knowledge is 'inside information'?" It could be said that perhaps a good majority don't. This could mean that we don't always use our ability to think consciously in what we

3

say or do. For example, we may have said or done things that on reflection we wish we hadn't. Exercise 1 offers an opportunity to self-reflect.

EXERCISE 1

Reflect on one occasion when you said or did something that you would have otherwise preferred not to have said or done.

Information obtained from Exercise 1 could be used to guide future behaviour, as it would appear that there is a price to pay for not implementing our ability to think consciously. As a health care practitioner one cannot afford to behave in a manner that is likely to cause harm or distress to those one is meant to help. Awareness of one's behaviour is crucial to any interaction but perhaps more so where these interactions involve patients. As Rungapadiachy (1999) states, self-awareness is a prerequisite skill for health care delivery. The implication is that health care practitioners would be in a much better position to empathise with their patients or clients. Moreover, the National Occupational Standards in Mental Health (2003) identifies 'practise in a reflective manner' as one of the key roles for mental health professionals. This notion could be extended to include all health care professionals. With this in mind, this chapter explores the concept of self-awareness with particular emphasis on how it can be used to establish effective relationships with patients and clients.

What is self-awareness?

According to Williams (2003), the use of the term self-awareness may be problematic in that each theorist and researcher may be focusing on a different construct when they refer to it. For example, self-awareness could be taken to mean 'a general self-knowledge (an ability to have insight into one's inner world and personality), but self-awareness has also been defined as a momentary state, such as self-consciousness' (Williams, 2003, p. 178). The momentary state of consciousness and its implication to care delivery will be discussed later in the section that deals with benefits and drawbacks of self-awareness. In an attempt to understand the concept of self-awareness, the notion of self is explored. However, the starting point is with an explanation of the word 'awareness'.

To be aware means to be conscious, sensitive, and alert. To be aware could also mean to know, recognise, and accept. According to Rawlins, Williams, and Beck (1993), awareness implies that an individual can focus his or her attention on a particular experience and promote 'individual "knowing" of that experience' (p. 30). Self-awareness therefore could be taken to mean focusing on self as well as, recognising, knowing, and accepting of self. An interesting point to note here is that people not only have an image of themselves but also know that this image is the object of the process of self-reflection (Hart & Fegley, 1994).

What is self?

The construct of self consists of all those descriptions that individuals ascribe to themselves. For example, these could include all self-representations that reflect how people see themselves. The words that I would use to describe myself would give some indications as to my sense of self. For example, whom I think and feel I am, my physical attributes, things that I do, and the various roles that I occupy would all form part of my sense of self. It could be argued that there is a further dimension to self in that these descriptive characteristics can also serve to modify an individual's sense of self to transform this particular individual in the desired direction (Demetriou, Kazi, & Georgiou, 1999). The implication is that self is significant in that it influences people's actual behaviour, motivation to initiate or disrupt activities, and feelings about themselves. For example, we may see ourselves as 'caring', and therefore we behave in a 'caring' way; however, interaction is perceived to come before thinking and self-reflection (Ashworth, 2003). The implications as pointed by Ashworth (2003) are two fold:

1. Inner thoughts and external communications are basically the same. Thoughts can be easily translated into words, and symbols form part of the interaction.

2. The capacity to reflect on one's own actions is an avenue for the formation of one's self-concept. Moreover, perceived feedback from others contributes to the ability to self-reflect.

According to James (1890), self is a hierarchical and multidimensional construct (see Figure 1.1). The two hierarchical levels are as follows:

1. The 'I-self' which is the 'knower' and includes all the observation and self-recording processes that generate the knowledge about ourselves. The 'I-self' is also referred to as the Knowing Self. In this instance self assumes the role of subject.

2. The 'me-self' is that knowledge we have about ourselves and is described as the sum of all that we call ours. The 'me-self' has at least three dimensions. These are

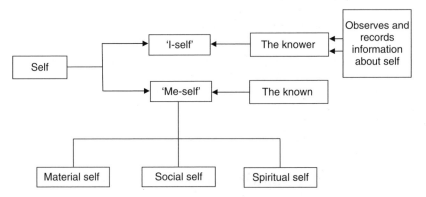

Figure 1.1 An overview of the hierarchical and multidimensional construct of self.

material self, social self, and spiritual self. The 'me-self' is also referred to as the known self and becomes the object.

Material self includes the representations of our bodies and possessions. The body is described as the innermost part of the material self. Moreover, certain parts of the body seem more intimately known to us than the rest (Hattie, 1992). Clothes, immediate family, homes, and possessions also form part of our material self. Social self is the recognition that we obtain from others such as friends and colleagues. According to James (1890), people generally have an innate tendency to get themselves noticed positively by others. Spiritual self is described as the inner or subjective being that contains the characteristics that are the most enduring and intimate parts of the self (Hattie, 1992). Spiritual self could be seen as reflective and involves people's thinking about themselves. Hence, Descartes' notion of 'I think, therefore I am'. The concepts of material self, social self, and spiritual self would be easier to relate to by engaging in Exercise 2.

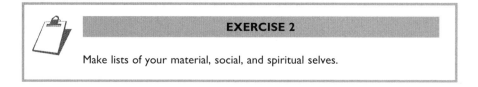

EXERCISE 2

Make lists of your material, social, and spiritual selves.

The process of gaining knowledge about ourselves almost seems as though we step out of ourself to observe ourself (see Figure 1.2). The end result of this observation is the 'me-self'. The act of stepping out of, looking at, observing, and recording oneself can be described as reflexivity. For Mead (1934), reflexivity means the turning back of one's experience upon oneself. James (1890) would argue that self-awareness is the conclusion that the 'I-self' arrives at to form the 'me-self'. In simple terms, if we are able to describe our material selves, our social selves, and our spiritual selves, we would, to some extent, be self-aware.

Self-awareness can be conceptualised both as a personality trait and a skill (Church, 1997). For example, Fletcher and Baldry (2000) state that trait self-awareness is found in a minority of individuals who could be described as being 'naturally' self-aware. This could mean that the majority of people would need to develop self-awareness as a skill. Self-awareness as a skill is related to factors influencing and biasing self-assessment. The implication is that learning to become self-aware would help to bring some element of objectivity in assessing oneself. The subjective self is therefore required to take on self as the object of one's own attention and thought.

Components of self-awareness

It could be said that there are at least three components to self-awareness and these are cognitive, affective, and behavioural. Cognitive refers to the mental process of comprehension. It includes memory, perception, past experience,

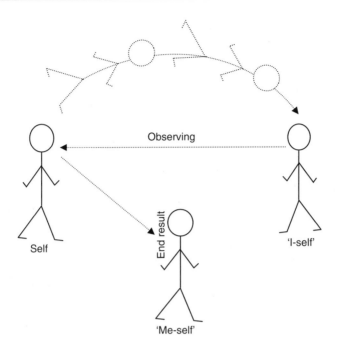

Figure 1.2 'I-self' is the observer and the 'me-self' becomes the end product of that observation.

expectation, appraisal, attribution, attitude, beliefs, and values. Moreover, these could be seen as the thinking aspect of an individual. Affective refers to the feeling aspect of self. Behavioural simply means the action that one engages in, and this could be verbal and/or non-verbal. There is a dynamic relationship between these three components in that thinking could affect feeling and behaviour, feeling could affect thinking and behaviour, and behaviour could affect thinking and feeling.

Cognitive self

The cognitive self could be described as the representations that we each have in our own minds of the kind of person we think we are. Exercise 3 attempts to clarify this point.

EXERCISE 3

Make a list of the kind of person you think you are. For example, how are you in company of others? Are you easy to get on with? Do you really listen when people speak with you? What are your beliefs about politicians? What are your strengths and weaknesses? The list is endless.

The conclusion that you would have drawn from Exercise 3 would indicate the representations of your cognitive self. However, Salzen (1998) argues that self-awareness is achieved through introspection that in itself is a conscious cognitive process. The implication is that cognitive knowledge about self cannot be objective. It could be argued that this realisation may in itself be helpful in that an individual may be able to guard against cognitive self-serving bias (see Chapter 7). Self-serving bias suggests the tendency to attribute positive events to self and negative events to external factors. For example, if we pass our exams it is because we are knowledgeable, but if we fail it is always because we have been unfairly marked. It could be argued that there may be some unconscious dynamics at play in the phenomenon of self-serving bias. This could also imply that we function at various depth of consciousness.

Levels of consciousness

According to Freud (1984), an individual has three levels of awareness and these are conscious, preconscious, and unconscious.

1. At a conscious level we have immediate access to materials. For example, at times we are aware that we are hungry. According to Epstein (1983), people have conscious theories of reality that include theories about themselves and the world.

2. At a preconscious level some thoughts and images are not in our immediate awareness, but we can access these with little or moderate effort. For example, we can try and bring to our awareness events of September 11, Tsunami, Live 8, and hurricane Katrina. Moreover, Epstein (1983) states that reactions at the preconscious level are often so automatic and fleeting that it may take special practice and training in order to be aware of certain preconscious thoughts and images. Epstein (1983) theorises that individuals use mental defence mechanisms[1] to shield them from awareness of their preconscious beliefs, thereby allowing them to deceive themselves into believing that their behaviour is more rational and less egocentric than is often the case.

3. At the unconscious level and 'under normal conditions' events are not available to our awareness. These may be for various reasons and one of which may be that such an event is morally unacceptable for the individual. Moreover, materials cannot be assimilated into the conscious system because they may be incongruous with that system. A typical example would be the repression of aggressive sexual impulses because of the incongruity between people's conception of their actual selves and their morally acceptable selves.[2] 'Expressed otherwise, not only do individuals repress, or dissociate, mental content because it contains taboo material that is guilt arousing, but they also dissociate mental content that threatens the stability or coherence of their overall conceptual systems' (Epstein, 1983, p. 231).

In summary, the cognitive self involves all descriptions, implicit or explicit, that people make of themselves in relation to their mental functions, abilities, strategies, and skills. In other words the cognitive self serves to judge self, others, and self in relation to others. Exercise 4 is an attempt to personalise cognitive self.

<table>
<tr><td>

EXERCISE 4

What do you think of the following groups of people?
Individuals who hear voices.
Individuals who are aggressive.
Individuals who harm themselves.
</td></tr>
</table>

What you think of the above individuals will indicate to some extent your judgement about them and hence one aspect of your cognitive self.

Emotive self

According to Salzen (1998), subjective emotions, like feelings of sensori-motor pleasure and displeasure, involve minimal cognitive processing and as such are believed to produce the objective observable display of emotion. It would appear that 'emotions are central to the recognition and acceptance of its existence' (Salzen, 1998, p. 300). The implication is that self-feeling is self-transparent. For example, generally speaking, an individual knows when he or she is feeling sad or happy,[3] and it would seem difficult to self-deny these feelings at a conscious level. However, Duval, Silva, and Lalwani (2001) conclude that both positive and negative effect can potentially induce self-awareness. For example, we feel happy when we are praised, and we become aware of this happy feeling. Similarly, we feel angry when we are insulted, and in some situations (as this is not always the case) we will be aware of this anger feeling.

Behavioural self

Most literature on self-awareness deal with its cognitive and affective aspects and very few if any address awareness of behaviour per se. This, to some extent, could be because behaviour includes the components of thinking and feeling. For example, when someone says 'let me think', this implies seeking the opportunity to engage in intellectual information processing. Thinking, therefore, becomes an act and as such a behaviour. Emotion, however, has three behavioural characteristics and these are physiological, expressive, and experiential. The physiological aspect of emotion is believed to have its roots in the limbic system of the brain. For example, arousal of particular parts of the limbic system leads to changes in heart rate, blood pressure, and increase in sweating. The expressive aspect of emotion is related to facial expression, vocal cues, and body movements. The experiential aspect of emotion is believed to be crucial to daily functioning in that it may be responsible for motivating action. For example, fear may be the motivation for escape, anger for attacking, and disgust for vomiting (Scherer & Ekman, 1984).

Based on Freud's (1984) notion of unconscious level of awareness it would seem that there are certain aspects of our behaviour that we are not aware of. This is evidenced in mental defence mechanisms that normally refer to unconscious strategies that we adopt in our attempt to deal with emotional conflicts. Mental defence mechanisms do not resolve conflicts as such, but they change the way we perceive or think about them. According to Smith, Nolen-Hoeksema, and Fredrickson (2003), mental defence mechanisms involve an element of self-deception. The basic and perhaps most important of all defence mechanisms is repression.

Repression

The essence of repression lies in turning something away, and keeping it at a distance, from the conscious. For example, memories and impulses that are too frightening, painful, and can evoke shame, guilt, or self-deprecation are often excluded from conscious awareness. Early evidence of repression is seen in Freud's notion of Oedipus (in boys) and Electra (in girls) complex. Freud believed that all young boys and girls have feelings of sexual attraction towards their opposite sex parent and feelings of rivalry and hostility towards their same sex parent. However, these impulses are blocked from consciousness in order to avoid the painful consequences of acting on them. In later life or adulthood people may repress feelings that are incongruous with their moral expectation and duty. For example, feeling of intense hate towards an intimate partner with murderous intention may be excluded from conscious awareness. It needs to be pointed out that repression is itself an unconscious act. Other defence mechanisms include suppression, regression, rationalisation, denial, projection, reaction formation, displacement, and introjection.

Suppression

Unlike repression, suppression is the conscious process of self-control where impulses and desires are kept at bay. This could be temporarily pushing aside memories that are likely to cause pain and/or discomfort. In its simplistic form a typical example could be putting one's financial problem aside while on holiday.

Regression

This is unconsciously adopting a behaviour that is appropriate to an earlier stage of development. Stage theorists like Freud (1973), Erickson (1963), and Piaget (1952) believe that an individual's personality develops in a series of stages from birth to maturity. From Freud's perspective, each stage of development brings with it some element of frustration and anxiety. If the levels of frustration and anxiety become too much, normal development may be temporarily or permanently halted. The child may remain fixed at the current stage. However, the intensity of frustration could be such that the resulting anxiety pushes that child into an earlier stage of development. For example, the child may revert back to thumb sucking or bed-wetting.

Rationalisation

One of the simplest explanations of rationalisation is through Aesop's fable of the fox and the sour grapes. The real reason the fox rejected the grapes was because it could not reach them but instead said that they were sour. The moral of this particular fable is that it is easy to despise the things that we cannot get.

Rationalisation is the unconscious process whereby a false but acceptable reason is offered for behaviour that has in fact a much less acceptable motive. Smith, Nolen-Hoeksema, and Fredrickson (2003) state that rationalisation serves two purposes. For example, it eases our disappointment when we fail to reach our goals and it provides us with acceptable motives for our behaviour. The overall aim is to place our behaviour in a more favourable light.

Denial

This is believed to occur when individuals are faced with an external reality that is too unpleasant to accept, for example the loss of an intimate partner or of a child. Denial and disbelief are often classed as the initial stage of bereavement (Kübler-Ross, 1969).[4] There would seem to be an unconscious refusal to accept that the loss has taken place or is imminent. Less severe forms of denial are seen in people who consistently ignore advice or whose marriage is failing but ignore all the signs.

Projection

In terms of projection 'I don't like you' becomes 'you don't like me'. When one's own unacceptable feeling is attributed to someone else, projection is said to be at play. For example, the child who dislikes his or her father may say 'my father hates me'.

Reaction formation

Adopting a behaviour opposite to that which reflects the individual's true feelings and intentions is seen as reaction formation. For example, an individual who may have negative feelings towards people of different ethnic origins campaigns actively for their rights. Similarly, someone who harbours sexual feeling for a member of the same sex may protest against homosexuality.

Displacement

This involves the transferring or shifting of emotion from a situation or object with which it is truly related to another target. Displacement is used when the real target is perceived as too threatening to confront directly. For example, our superior tells us off and we in turn take it out on our subordinates. Kicking the door is perhaps the simplest example.

Introjection

This is a process whereby an individual takes on the values or personal attributes of a significant other and behaves as though these are really his or her own. For example, we may have no qualms about sex before marriage but our parents condemn it. This leads to a conflict of values. However, because of our emotional ties and not wishing to displease them, we take on their values and behave as though we too condemn sex before marriage. Exercises 5 and 6 help to develop the concept of defence mechanism as applied to self and others.

EXERCISE 5

Using a similar format as in Table 1.1, identify an appropriate example (from personal experience) in each of the mental defence mechanisms listed below.

Table 1.1 Defence mechanisms as related to self

Defence mechanism	Self
Repression	
Suppression	
Rationalisation	
Denial	
Projection	
Reaction formation	
Displacement	
Introjection	

EXERCISE 6

Identify an appropriate example in each of the mental defence mechanisms listed below from your observation of patients (for example, how might patients exhibit relevant defence mechanisms).

Table 1.2 Defence mechanisms as related to patients

Defence mechanism	Others as in patient
Repression	
Suppression	
Rationalisation	
Denial	
Projection	
Reaction formation	
Displacement	
Introjection	

Forms of self-awareness

According to Neisser (1997), self-awareness is based on five distinct forms of information and these are as follows.

Ecological self-awareness

Ecological self-awareness suggests that individuals have to have the ability to process information regarding their immediate physical environment. According to Leary and Buttermore (2003), as individuals move through their environment, they experience visual, auditory, and other cues that are intimately linked to their bodily positions and movements. They would thus conclude that they are in the here and now and engaging in a specific activity.

Interpersonal self-awareness

Interpersonal self-awareness refers to people recognising that they are in fact interacting with others at a particular place and time. Neisser (1988) argues that the nature, direction, timing, and intensity of people's interaction with one another shows that they have a sophisticated knowledge about themselves and their ongoing behaviour that allows them to self-regulate effectively in ongoing social encounters. Interpersonal self-awareness therefore could be taken to mean knowing how to behave in social situation. Social intelligence would encapsulate interpersonal self-awareness and will be discussed later in the chapter.

Extended self-awareness

Extended self-awareness consists of thoughts about oneself in the past and in the future. For example, 'I am today the same person who did thus-and-so last year or who will do this-or-that next week' (Leary & Buttermore, 2003, p. 368). The extended self-awareness allows the individual to think about himself or herself in other times and places. This involves the act of reflection and forward thinking.

Private self-awareness

Private self-awareness as the phrase suggests involves processing private, subjective information including thoughts, feelings, intentions, and other states that are not available to other people. Private self-awareness allows people to reflect on their subjective experience. The resulting information is used to anticipate personal reaction to future events with the knowledge that other people are not privileged to that information. According to Leary and Buttermore (2003), private self-awareness may underlie people's ability to infer other people's states. For example, in order to understand and predict other people's reactions we may make reference to our own inner states. 'We infer others' feelings, intentions, and attitudes, for example, by extrapolating from our own (with adjustments based on knowledge about the other person), thus requiring the capacity for private self-reflection' (Leary & Buttermore, 2003, p. 381).

Conceptual self-awareness

Conceptual self-awareness (seen as synonymous with the symbolic self) involves labels, traits, categories, and roles that we use to conceptualise ourselves, for example lecturers and students (Leary & Buttermore, 2003). However, conceptual self-awareness also has an evaluative function. The implication is that people may categorise themselves as good or bad and effective or ineffective.

Conceptual self-awareness serves to provide an individual with an identity and self-concept.

Self-concept

According to Hattie (1992), self-conceptions are individuals' cognitive appraisals of their attributes. However, these are the more private aspects of themselves. Self-concept refers to a particular cluster of ideas and attitudes that we have about ourselves at any given moment. The implication is that self-concept is not static, and it can change. According to Adler (1963), self-concept is both the artist and the picture. This suggests that individuals are able to self-reflect in order to know that they know what they know about themselves. However, some people have more reflexivity than others. Hence, some know more about themselves than others. It could be argued that self-concept is not merely what we know about ourselves but involves the relationship between what we know and how we behave. For example, our self-concept may guide our behaviour (this point will be discussed later). According to Hamacheck (1992), self-concept has at least four components and these are physical, social, emotional, and intellectual. These components are displayed in the way we describe ourselves. For example, we may feel and think that

- our nose is too big (physical self-concept)
- we are approachable and friendly (social self-concept)
- we are happy (emotional self-concept)
- we are knowledgeable (intellectual self-concept).

These four components are interrelated in that conclusions drawn from one will influence the others. For example, 'big nose' implies that we are not happy with it and perhaps wish to have a smaller nose. We may as a result feel depressed and our approachability and friendliness may disappear. We may even see ourselves as less intelligent. The implication is that these clusters (physical, social, emotional, and intellectual) contribute to form a general self-concept, and for this reason self-concept is described as hierarchical (Shavelson, Hubner, & Stanton, 1976) (see Figure 1.3).

On closer analysis two principal sub-themes seem to emerge from these clusters. These are self-image and self-esteem. It is worthwhile noting that in some instances self-concept and self-image have been used interchangeably (Petersen, 1981). However, in the context of this chapter self-image is taken to mean a view of what one looks like on the outside, for example, one's body image. These sub-themes are evaluated against the self that we would like to be, that is our ideal self. This result is in our self-esteem.

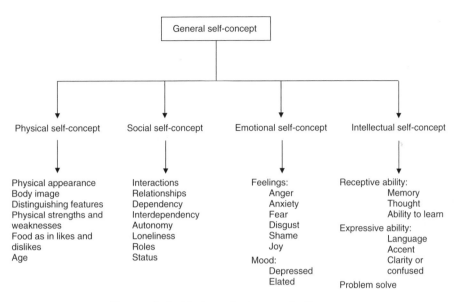

Figure 1.3 The hierarchical nature of self-concept.

Body image, ideal-self, and self-esteem

It could be argued that one of the key features of physical self-concept is our body image. Described as a multifaceted psychological experience of embodiment, especially but not exclusively one's physical appearance (Cash, 2004), body image is significant to one's general self-concept. For example, our life experiences are influenced by the body we happen to occupy. Our body is also seen as the tool for actions and interactions. The attitude we hold towards our body will reflect our identity and the way we present ourselves to others. Appearance matters to most of us; moreover, 'Individuals' own subjective experiences of their appearance were often even more psychologically powerful than the objective or social "reality" of their appearance' (Cash, 2004, p. 1). However, it could be argued that it is not what we look like that matters but instead the way we think and feel about our looks. The implication is that body image has two distinct poles and these are positive and negative. Exercise 7 serves to personalise the concept of body image.

EXERCISE 7

What do you like and dislike about your physical appearance?

It is possible to work out whether you have a positive or negative body image based on your answer in Exercise 7. It could be said that our interpretations of our physical appearances are sometimes dependent on our interpretation of others. For example, we may think our noses are too big but we may also feel that it is not as big as the next person. In this instance, we may take comfort that there is someone worse off than us. This could mean keeping the negative evaluation of our physical attributes in check.

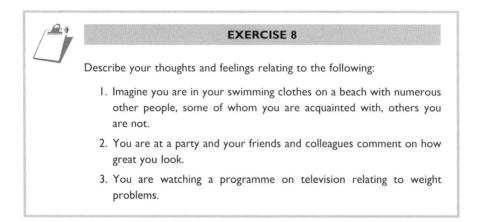

EXERCISE 8

Describe your thoughts and feelings relating to the following:

1. Imagine you are in your swimming clothes on a beach with numerous other people, some of whom you are acquainted with, others you are not.

2. You are at a party and your friends and colleagues comment on how great you look.

3. You are watching a programme on television relating to weight problems.

Emerging issues for discussion in Exercise 8 relate to who you are and how you feel about your body. Evidence suggests that obese and overweight people are more likely to have a negative body image (Cash & Roy, 1999). However, it would seem that the more we accept and like our bodies, the more secure we will feel and the less anxious we are likely to be. However, if the gap between our self-image and ideal self (the self or attributes that we would like to possess) is wide and unbridgeable this could lead to a low self-esteem. For example, if we see ourselves completely different to the person we would like to be (or the attributes that we would like to have) and we are not able to change, we may suffer mental health problems characterised by low self-esteem. Self-esteem can be described as the value one holds of oneself, and this is contingent on one's successes and failures. Success in one's life may contribute to high self-esteem, whereas failure may result in low self-esteem.

Factors influencing self-concept formation

It could be said that self-concept is learned and that its development emerges out of an individual's interaction with significant others. Significant others include parents, teachers, friends, and peers. Therefore, self as such does not exist at birth. According to Rogers (1959), newborn babies perceive all their experiences as a unitary whole and do not have the capacity to differentiate between themselves and the environment. The process of self-concept formation starts the moment infants are able to distinguish between themselves and the external world. For Piaget (1952), self-concept formation begins during the first phase of development known as the sensorimotor stage. It becomes clear that the initial years of development are crucial to the formation of self-concept. Moreover, parents have the greatest impact on the developing self-concept for preschool children (Burns, 1982). However, Rogers (1951) argues that one of the factors influencing self-concept formation is the universal need for positive regard. The implication is that everyone has a desire to be loved and accepted by significant others. Rogers (1951) argues that a child's self-concept is governed by his or her organismic valuing process, whereby each new experience is evaluated in terms of whether it facilitates or impedes his or her psychological growth and development. For example, the experience of hunger, thirst, cold, pain, and loud noises hinder growth, whereas food, water, security, and love promote it. However, the need for love and acceptance is so intense that children are generally prepared to sacrifice their organismic valuing process to satisfy their need for positive regard (see Chapter 9). Hence, they unconsciously employ the mental defence mechanism of introjection. Moreover, children also learn that certain types of behaviour lend themselves to positive regard and other types do not. Positive regard that are dependent on good behaviour are called conditions of worth. When positive regard is dependent on conditions of worth, this is called conditional positive regard. Rogers (1951) argues that both conditions of worth and conditional positive regards are detrimental to a child's psychological growth and development. It could be said therefore that positive self-concept emerges out of unconditional positive regard. The implication is that people should be praised for who they are and not on whether what they do pleases us.

Becoming and developing self-awareness

Reflecting on Hamachek's (1992) sentiment, if we want to know ourselves, then we need to observe what others are doing. If we want to understand others, then we need to search within ourselves. However,

> Most of us are inclined to do exactly the opposite. We observe the other person to understand him or her, and we probe within ourselves to understand ourselves better. Normally, we look at the other person objectively; we behold their flaws, weaknesses, self-deceptions, and even their prejudices masquerading as principles. When we probe within ourselves, however, we are not inclined to see the same personal distortions. What we "see" are our good intentions, our noblest ambitions, the fine deeds we have performed, and the sacrifices we have made.
>
> (Hamachek, 1992, p. 318)

The implication is that we use one pair of glasses to look at ourselves and a different pair to look at others. We also seem to be much more critical of others than we are of ourselves. The reason as Hamachek (1992) says is that it may not be so much that we are deliberately setting out to deceive ourselves but instead we are trying to view a picture from inside the frame. A point that has already been made is that in order to see ourselves as we truly are, we need to step out of and observe ourselves. Although a start, however, we are not guaranteed to see all there is to see. 'We can meditate for hours or analyze ourselves for weeks and not progress an inch farther–any more than we can smell our own breath or laugh when we tickle ourselves no matter how hard we try' (Hamachek, 1992, p. 318). This suggests that reflexivity on its own is not adequate for self-understanding. One possible solution rests with Adler's (1964) notion of social feeling. Possessing social feeling implies that one has gone beyond one's own private experiences, motives, and thoughts in order to understand the needs and goals of others. The principal sentiment here is to be less self-preoccupied and more attentive to what others are going through. This would serve as an avenue for self-knowledge. For example, it may never have dawned on us that someone needs help until we see our neighbours running to help. Similarly, a person saying 'I wish my partner would do more in the house' could serve as a cue for us to realise that we should pull our weight. Other ways of self-knowledge could be through what has been described as the dynamics between trust-disclosure-feedback (see Rungapadiachy, 1999, Chapter 18). The argument is that the more able we are to trust someone, the more we will self-disclose and the more objective the feedback will be when we ask for it. In summary, we could enhance our self-awareness skills by

- reflexivity

- keeping journals

- observing what others do

- listening to what others are saying

- trust-disclosure-feedback

- instructions to focus on personal thoughts and feelings as in the exercises suggested throughout this chapter. This could also be seen as guided memory recall.

Benefits and drawbacks of self-awareness

According to Duval and Wicklund (1972), when people are self-aware their consciousness is focused on their thoughts and feelings, their personal history, their body, or other personal aspects of themselves. Being self-aware in principle means that we should be more calculated in what we do. For example, if we are aware that what we do is offensive to some people, then we may think twice before exhibiting such behaviour. It could be argued therefore that self-awareness serves as an adaptive function principally in the form of self-control. According to Salzen (1998), 'the function of self-awareness then, at the full cognitive level, is not to allow the luxury of introspection but as a mechanism or device for the integration of personal and social behaviour into a single learned self-controlling system' (p. 308). For example, being aware of a socially unattractive mannerism such as farting or scratching one's private parts in the company of others should in theory contribute to their eradication. Moreover, Gallup (1998) calls this a sense of personal agency that emerges as a result of interacting and informally experimenting with both animate and inanimate features in our environment. For example, we learn that what we do, when we do it, and how we do it has an influence on the outcome.

According to Vorauer and Ross (1999), people should be more inclined to see their own actions as conveying information congruent with their personal attributes and attitudes when they are self-aware. For example, I would come to see myself as a confident lecturer in the way I deliver my lectures. Outside, observers are expected to see this as well. This suggests an element of deliberate communication. Leary and Buttermore (2003) argue that deliberate communication requires the communicator to infer how the audience is likely to react to various communicative acts. The implication is that self-awareness may underpin our ability to infer other people's states. Moreover, as Leary and Buttermore (2003) state, there seems to be no way to understand and predict other people's reaction except with reference to our inner states. 'We could, in effect, imagine what it's like to be them, because we know what it's like to be ourselves' (Humphrey, 1986, p. 71). Vorauer and Ross (1999) found that increased self-awareness is associated with feelings of transparency. The notion of transparency suggests our beliefs about the extent to which our personal qualities can be accurately perceived from our behaviour. However, dwelling on ourselves as objects can make us aware of how we fall short of our ideals thus leading us to conclude negative views of ourselves (Duval & Wicklund, 1972). Moreover, this may explain why according to Maslow (1968) some people are reluctant to engage in self-awareness activities.

Interestingly, being self-aware is not without its drawbacks. For example, verbal disfluencies among stutterers have been attributed to self-awareness (Mullen, Migdal, & Rozell, 2003). The implication is that stutters are compounded by self-awareness. One argument is that the more aware individuals are of their stutters the more pronounced the stutters become. Moreover, Williams and Hill (1996) found that when novice therapists were aware of their own negative self-talk, they also reported feeling more negative about their overall therapeutic performance and about their clients' reactions. Williams (2003) found that momentary states of heightened therapist self-awareness may be hindering the process of therapy. For example, the more anxious the therapists were before a session, the more they focused on themselves during the session. Therapist momentary self-awareness was negatively related to clients' perception of therapists' helpfulness. Williams (2003) suggests that higher amounts of momentary self-awareness in therapists may be distracting to the helping process. Similarly, the more aware we are of our anxieties, for example, before presenting at a conference, the more exaggerated our anxieties may become.

Self-awareness and engaging with patients

It could be argued that the benefits of being self-aware far outweigh its drawbacks. It is worth noting that self-awareness on its own cannot not guarantee effective engagement. However, self-awareness in the hands of a skilled practitioner would significantly improve the quality of engagement. For example, Schwebel and Coster (1998) suggest that self-awareness is a fundamental characteristic in a well-functioning practitioner. Moreover, self-awareness is also one of the primary principles of ethical practice (Rubin, 2000). As McLeod (2003) states, caring for patients involves empathic listening and awareness of the needs and feelings of the patient as well as one's own. 'Too often we lead unbalanced lives in terms of work, relationships, play, and personal time. We frequently strive for perfection, deny our needs and feelings, assume total responsibility for the patients, and are altruistic to the point of self-denial' (McLeod, 2003, p. 2135). It seems clear from literature that health care practitioners' self-awareness is central to care delivery. For example, Severinsson (2001) posits that the degree to which practitioners are aware of their views of human beings and of a caring philosophy can be crucial for the care provided. What seems obvious is that self-awareness does contribute positively to health care delivery. In order to explain how self-awareness can be applied to health care practice we would need to revisit the five distinct areas of awareness: ecological, interpersonal, extended, private, and conceptual. The principal sentiment that can be deduced from these is that one has sensory acuity of one's physical environment, interactions with others, thoughts (as in past, present, and future), much more private and subjective feelings and thinking, and who one is. Once we are equipped with these areas of awareness, we would then have to extrapolate how it feels to be someone else but more specifically how it must feel to be in need of health care services. Successful engagement with patients is underpinned by three prerequisite skills that would enable practitioners to use self as agents of therapeutic interventions and these are empathic understanding, social intelligence, and emotional intelligence.

Empathic understanding

According to Nelson-Jones (2000), empathic understanding is another term for empathy. Empathy can be described as a form of emotional knowing or the experiencing of another person's feeling. Moreover, Rogers (1957) states that empathy is the sensing of another person's private world *as if* it were one's own, but without losing the 'as if' quality. The implication is that the practitioner would need to 'get into the shoes' of their patients in order to understand their private subjective world. Raskin and Rogers (1989) suggest that when 'empathy is at its best, the two individuals are participating in a process which may be compared to that of a couple dancing, the client leading, the therapist following: the smooth, spontaneous back-and-forth flow of energy in the interaction has its own aesthetic rhythm' (Raskin & Rogers, 1989, p. 157). However, Raskin and Rogers warned that if one thinks empathy is just about repeating the client's words, one is horribly mistaken. Empathy is seen as an interaction in which the practitioner is a warm, sensitive, respectful companion in the typically difficult exploration of the client's emotional world. Rogers (1959) argues that empathic understanding takes place when the practitioner is able to capture the patient's feelings, emotions, and thoughts through his or her words and action. Moreover, based on the practitioner's own experiences, thoughts, and feelings he or she communicates to the clients those feelings that were verbally expressed by the latter. In summary, when practitioners are able to demonstrate their ability to appreciate their patients' phenomenological world, they would be described as having 'empathic understanding'. Exercise 9 helps to clarify your own position about the notion of empathy.

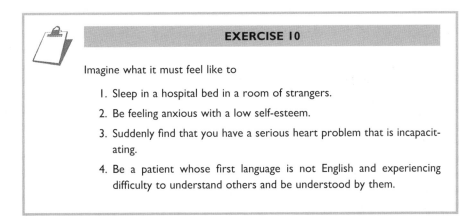

EXERCISE 9

Is it possible to empathise with another person? If so how might you achieve this?

According to Berlo (1960), one school of thought argues that there is no such thing as empathy. The implication is that one could never truly empathise with another person. This argument is based on the notion that it is impossible to 'get into' another person's world, feel it, and sense it just as the other person would. From a personal perspective, I feel it may be difficult to empathise with another person but not impossible. As Berlo (1960) states, the development of empathy requires a special kind of talent. One could argue that effective listening, attending, and responding could help practitioners to develop empathic understanding. However, it does mean that practitioners would have to do their homework, and this would involve getting to know patients' personal and medical history and listen to what they have to say. Most importantly, ask yourself the following question. 'How might it feel to be, for example, depressed or anxious?' Therefore, another prerequisite for the caring process is for practitioners to have a good understanding of patients' complaints. This would serve as an avenue to attempt to enter the patient's world. Exercise 10 may help to enhance the use of self-awareness in your clinical practice.

EXERCISE 10

Imagine what it must feel like to

1. Sleep in a hospital bed in a room of strangers.
2. Be feeling anxious with a low self-esteem.
3. Suddenly find that you have a serious heart problem that is incapacitating.
4. Be a patient whose first language is not English and experiencing difficulty to understand others and be understood by them.

This type of reflection could be linked with extended self-awareness, for example, imagining oneself in a different time and environment with different health status. This would serve to create a much more genuine relationship when engaging with patients. Moreover, it could be argued that using one's own experience to make inferences about the experiences of others could also serve to reinforce one's ability to become socially and emotionally intelligent.

Social intelligence

Social intelligence can be described as a by-product of self-awareness (Gallup, 1998), hence the need for introspection and reflection in order to understand one's intrapersonal and interpersonal dynamics. Social intelligence has its origin in the work of Thorndike (1920), who describes it as one's ability to understand and manage relationships with others. According to Vernon (1933), to be socially intelligent means to possess the ability to get on with people in general as well as in social situation. This implies that one must have knowledge of social matters and have insight into the temporary moods or underlying personality traits of people. For Egan (1977), social intelligence means knowing what to do in interpersonal situations. Implicit within any definition of social intelligence is the essence of being able to evaluate with reasonable accuracy the social responses and expectations of others. One could argue that the skill to predict other people's social responses is an integral part of daily living. In fact, according to the social intelligence hypothesis the need to cope with complex social relationships, acquire and manage social knowledge in order to predict responses of group members was 'a decisive factor in the evolution of human intelligence' (Dautenhahn, 1998, p. 577). It would be erroneous to assume that every human being is socially intelligent just the same as it would be incorrect to believe that we are all cognitively intelligent. However, as agents of health care delivery, being socially intelligent is a prerequisite. Moreover, practitioners must develop a 'natural feel' for people. For example, when interacting with patients, practitioners would need to show understanding, sensitivity in their interaction, as well as respecting the needs and wishes of the former. According to Sternberg (1985), implicit within social intelligence is the concept of managerial intelligence. The implication is that health service practitioners not only need to understand others but they must also know how to cope with their patients' behaviour. In summary, the principal characteristics of social intelligence include being aware of and sensitive to the needs of patients as in demonstrating empathic understanding and engaging in effective interpersonal communication. For example, we need to know WHAT to say, WHEN to say it, WHERE to say it, HOW to say it, and WHOM to say it.

Emotional intelligence

Coined by Salovey and Mayer (1990) the concept of emotional intelligence was initially defined as 'the ability to monitor one's own feeling and emotions, to discriminate among them, and to use this information to guide one's thinking and actions' (p. 189). Reflecting on this and other definitions, Mayer and Salovey (1997) feel that emotional intelligence is much more than how it was first conceptualised. They revised their original thoughts to incorporate four principal themes in their definition and these are perception, appraisal, and expression of emotion; emotional facilitation of thinking; understanding and analysing emotions as well as employing emotional knowledge; and reflective regulation of emotions to promote emotional and intellectual growth. The attributes of each of the four themes are highlighted below.

■ **Perceive accurately, appraise, and express emotion**: This theme implies that emotionally intelligent individuals have the ability to recognise their own and those of other people's emotions through physical states as well as feelings (physical sensations) and thoughts. For example, given that we are emotionally intelligent, we should be able to recognise by facial expressions, how sad, happy, or angry patients look like. Similarly, we should be able to recognise the physical sensations that we are feeling. Mayer and Salovey (1997) state that the emotion and feeling as experienced by self can be generalised onto others through imaginative thinking. You would have already had a flavour of the notion of imaginative thinking in Exercise 10 where you are asked to imagine how it must feel to be, for example, anxious. The argument here is that being already aware of how it feels to be anxious you would use this feeling as a template to recognise when other people are anxious. The ability to recognise false or manipulative expression of emotion in others is a further characteristic of emotional intelligence.

■ **Access and/or generate feelings when they facilitate thought**: The implication in this theme is that emotions prioritise thinking by directing attention to important information (Mayer & Salovey, 1997). Emotionally intelligent people would not allow their worries to spoil the day. Instead, they would actively address the issue. For example, knowing that one has to meet a deadline, one would not sit and worry about it. Instead, one would start prioritising what needs to be done and set about doing it. Emotionally intelligent individuals will therefore engage in a problem-solving approach. Moreover, emotions are readily accessible and serve as a template to help in evaluating feelings. For example, we may know from personal experience how changes affect us. Therefore, we can choose whether or not to engage in events that require us to make changes. In this instance we would have used our past emotional experience to direct future behaviour. Implicit within this theme is the ability to recognise that one's mood influences one's perspective on objects or events. Mayer and Salovey (1997) call it mood congruent judgement. The implication is that good mood leads to optimism (there is light at the end of the tunnel) and bad mood to pessimism (no, its an on coming train). Moreover, emotional states dictate the strategy that one adopts in solving problems. For example, we would behave differently when we are in a good mood in comparison to when we are in a bad mood.

■ **Understand and analyse emotions and employ emotional knowledge**: This theme deals with the understanding of emotion and application of emotional knowledge in future behaviour. The development of emotional recognition starts in childhood where the child learns to label emotions through interaction with significant others. Mayer and Salovey (1997) state that parents teach children about emotional reasoning by linking emotions to situations. For example, the child learns that a frustrating situation can lead to anger; loss leads to sadness; and so on. The implication is that emotionally intelligent individuals should be able to recognise and understand the relationship between events and emotional expression. Moreover, they should recognise the complexity of the experience of emotion in that it is possible to experience more than one emotion at the same time, for example, anger and anticipation, fear and surprise, sadness and relief, and so on. The employment of emotional knowledge in future behaviour could be in the form of 'an individual who feels unlovable might reject another's care for fear of later rejection' (Mayer & Salovey, 1997, p. 14).

- **Reflective regulation of emotions to promote emotional and intellectual growth**: The implication for emotionally intelligent practitioners is that they should be able to accept the expression of emotions regardless of whether these are pleasant or unpleasant. In fact, Mayer and Salovey believe that emotional reaction should be welcomed. However, one needs to know when to withdraw from an emotionally charged situation. Moreover, emotionally intelligent practitioner should have the ability to monitor and manage emotions in self and in others. It could be argued that emotional growth can only take place when negative emotions are moderated and pleasant ones are enhanced without any attempt to repress or exaggerate the information that they communicate.

Summary

Possessing and recognising a wealth of self-knowledge is the key to the making of an effective health practitioner. The importance of self-awareness on the part of health care practitioners and its pivotal role need to be acknowledged. Self, as was discussed, is made up of the 'I-self' (the knower) and the 'me-self' (the known). The implication is that the 'I-self' becomes the observer of self and the end product is the 'me-self'. Awareness is the consciousness of an event and in the context of this chapter, this relates to cognitive, affective, and behavioural aspects of self. Five distinct forms of self-awareness are highlighted as ecological, interpersonal, extended, private, and conceptual. Conceptual self-awareness contributes to the formation of one's identity and self-concept. Self-concept was described as consisting of at least four themes highlighted as physical, social, emotional, and intellectual. Self-concept formation is said to be learned and that its development occurs as a result of interaction with significant others. Moreover, parents are reported to have the greatest impact on the developing child's self-concept. One of the key ingredients for the development of a positive conception of self rests with the notion of unconditional positive regards. The implication is that the developing child would not have to go to the extreme of displaying introjection in order to be praised. The principal sentiment that is conveyed throughout is that self-awareness is a prerequisite for health service delivery. Some practitioners may possess the trait of self-awareness; however, most of us need to learn to be self-aware and one of the ways is through reflexivity. Interestingly, being self-aware does have some drawbacks but one would still maintain that these are few and far between. From what has been presented so far, the common element between the three core skills for a helping relationship (that is, empathic understanding, social intelligence, and emotional intelligence) is self-awareness. For example, empathic understanding suggests possessing knowledge of the feeling of the other person as well as conveying this knowledge to him or her (see Chapter 9, perceived empathic understanding). Social intelligence means to know the what, when, where, and how of interactions. Emotional intelligence is having the ability to monitor one's own feeling and emotions, to discriminate among them, and to use this information to guide one's thinking and actions. In order to be able to do these one needs to be self-aware. Social intelligence has already been described as a by-product of self-awareness. The same could be said for both empathic understanding and emotional intelligence.

References

Adler, A. (1963). *Understanding Human Nature*. Translated by Walter Béran Wolfe. London: Allen & Unwin.

Adler, A. (1964). *Social Interest: A Challenge to Mankind*. New York: Capricorn Books.

Ashworth, P. (2003). The origins of qualitative psychology. In J. A. Smith (ed.), *Qualitative Psychology: A Practical Guide to Research Method* (pp. 4–24). London, Thousand Oaks, and New Delhi: Sage Publications.

Berlo, D. K. (1960). *The Process of Communication: An Introduction to Theory and Practice*. New York: Holt, Rinehart, and Winston.

Burns, R. B. (1982). *Self-Concept Development and Education*. London: Holt, Rinehart, and Winston.

Cash, T. (2004). Body image: past, present, and future. *Body Image*, 4(1), 1–5.

Cash, T. F. and Roy, R. E. (1999). Pounds of flesh: weight, gender, and body images. In J. Sobal and D. Maurer (eds.), *Interpreting Weight: The Social Management of Fatness and Thinness* (pp. 209–228). Hawthorne: Aldine de Gruyter.

Church, A. H. (1997). Do you see what I see? An exploration of congruence in ratings form multiple perspectives. *Journal of Applied Social Psychology*, 27, 983–1020.

Dautenhahn, K. (1998). The art of designing socially intelligent agents: science, fiction, and the human in the loop. *Applied Artificial Intelligence*, 12, 573–617.

Demetriou, A., Kazi, S., and Georgiou, S. (1999). The emerging self: the convergence of mind, personality and thinking styles. *Developmental Science*, 21(4), 387–422.

Duval, T. S., Silva, P., and Lalwani, N. (2001). *Self-Awareness and Causal Attribution: A Dual Systems Theory*. Boston: Dordrecht and London: Kluwer Academic Publishers.

Duval, S. and Wicklund, R. A. (1972). *A Theory of Self-Awareness*. New York: Academic Press.

Egan, G. (1977). *You & Me: The Skills of Communicating and Relating to Others*. Monterey: Brooks/Cole Publishing Company.

Epstein, S. (1983). The unconscious, the preconscious, and the self-concept. In J. Suls and A. G. Greenwald (eds.), *Psychological Perspectives on The Self* (Vol. 2, pp. 219–247). Hillsdale and London: Lawrence Erlbaum Associate Publishers.

Erickson, H. (1963). *Childhood and Society*. New York: Norton.

Fletcher, C. and Baldry, C. (2000). A study of individual differences and self-awareness in the context of multi-source feedback. *Journal of Occupational and Organizational Psychology*, 73, 303–319.

Freud, S. (1973). *Introductory Lectures on Psychoanalysis*. London: Penguin Books.

Freud, S. (1984). *On Metapsychology*. London: Penguin Books.

Gallup, G. G. (1998). Self-awareness and the evolution of social intelligence. *Behavioural Processes*, 42, 239–247.

Hamachek, D. (1992). *Encounters with Self*. Fort Worth, New York, London, Sydney, and Tokyo: Harcourt Brace Jovanovich College Publishers.

Hart, H. and Fegley, S. (1994). Social imitation and the emergence of a mental model of self. In S. T. Parker, R. W. Mitchell, and M. L. Boccia (eds.), *Self-Awareness in Animals and Humans: Developmental Perspectives*. Cambridge: Cambridge University Press.

Hattie, J. (1992). *Self-Concept*. Hillsdale: Hove. L. Earlbaum Associates.

Humphrey, N. (1986). *The Inner Eye*. London: Faber and Faber.

James, W. (1890). *Principles of Psychology*. Chicago: Encyclopaedia Britannica.

Kübler-Ross, E. (1969). *On Death and Dying*. London: Routledge.

Leary, M. R. and Buttermore, N. R. (2003). The evolution of the human self: tracing the natural history of self-awareness. *Journal for the Theory of Social Behaviour*, 33(4), 365–404.

Maslow, A. H. (1968). *Towards a Psychology or Being*. New York: Van Nostrand.

Mayer, J. D. and Salovey, P. (1997). What is emotional intelligence? In P. Salovey and D. J. Sluyter (eds.), *Emotional Development and Emotional Intelligence* (pp. 3–31). New York: Basic Books.

McLeod, M. (2003). The caring physician: a journey in self-exploration and self-care. *The American Journal of Gastroenterology*, 98(10), 2135–2138.

Mead, G. H. (1934). *Mind, Self and Society: From the Standpoint of a Social Behaviourist*. Chicago: The University of Chicago Press.

Mullen, B., Migdal, M., and Rozell, D. (2003). Self-awareness, deindividuation, and social identity: unravelling theoretical paradoxes by filling empirical lacunae. *Personality and Social Psychology Bulletin*, 29(9), 1071–1081.

National Occupational Standards in Mental Health (2003). *Unit A1: Develop your own Knowledge and Practice*. Available at http://www.skillsforhealth.org.uk/page/competences/completed-competences-projects/list/mental-health?id=62.

Neisser, U. (1988). Five kinds of self knowledge. *Philosophical Psychology*, 1, 35–59.

Neisser, U. (1997). The roots of self-knowledge: Perceiving self, I, it, and thou. In J. G. Snodgrass and R. L. Thompson (eds.), *The Self Across Psychology* (pp. 19–33). New York: New York Academy of Sciences.

Nelson-Jones, R. (2000). *Six Key Approaches to Counselling and Therapy*. London and New York: Continuum.

Piaget, J. (1952). *The Origins of Intelligence in Children*. London: Routledge and Kagan Paul.

Petersen, D. M. (1981). The development of self-concept in adolescence. In M. D. Lynch, A. A. Norem-Bebeisen, and K. J. Gurgen (eds.), *Self-Concept: Advances in Theory and Research* (pp. 191–218). Cambridge: Ballinger.

Raskin, N. J. and Rogers, C. R. (1989). Person-centered therapy. In R. J. Corsini and D. Wedding (eds.), *Current Psychotherapies* (pp. 155–194). Itasca: F. E. Peacock Publishers, Inc.

Rawlins, R. P., Williams, S. R., and Beck, C. K. (1993). *Mental Health Psychiatric Nursing: A Holistic Life-Cycle Approach*. St. Louis, London, Sydney, and Toronto: Mosby Year Book, Inc.

Rogers, C. R. (1951). *Client-Centred Therapy: Its Current Practice, Implications, and Theory*. Boston: Houghton Mifflin Company.

Rogers, C. R. (1957). The necessary and sufficient conditions of therapeutic personality change. *Journal of Consulting Psychology*, 21, 95–103.

Rogers, C. R. (1959). A theory of therapy, personality and interpersonal relationships, as developed in the client-centered framework. In S. Koch (ed.), *Psychology: A Study of Science* (pp. 184–256). New York: McGraw Hill.

Rubin, S. (2000). Differentiating multiple relationships from multiple dimensions of involvement: therapeutic space at the interface of client, therapist, and society. *Psychotherapy: Theory, Research, Practice, Training*, 37, 315–324.

Rungapadiachy, D. M. (1999). *Interpersonal Communication and Psychology for Health Care Professional: Theory and Practice*. Oxford: Butterworth/Heinemann.

Salovey, P. and Mayer, J. D. (1990). Emotional Intelligence. *Imagination, Cognition, and Personality*, 9(3), 185–211.

Salzen, E. (1998). Emotion and self-awareness. *Applied Animal Behaviour Science*, 57, 299–313.

Scherer, K. R. and Ekman, P. (1984). *Approaches to Emotion*. Hillsdale and London: L. Erlbaum Associate.

Schwebel, M. and Coster, J. (1998). Well-functioning in professional psychologists: as program heads see it. *Professional Psychology: Research & Practice*, 29, 284–292.

Severinsson, E. I. (2001). Confirmation, meaning and self-awareness as core concepts of the nursing supervision model. *Nursing Ethics*, 2001, 8(1), 36–44.

Shavelson, R. J., Hubner, J. J., and Stanton, G. C. (1976). Self-concept: validation of construct interpretations. *Review of Educational Research*, 46, 407–441.

Smith, E. E., Nolen-Hoeksema, S., and Fredrickson, B. (2003). *Atkinson and Hilgard's Introduction to psychology*. Belmont and London: Wadsworth.

Sternberg, R. J. (1985). *Beyond IQ*. New York: Cambridge University Press.

Thorndike, E. L. (1920). Intelligence and its uses. *Harper's Magazine*, 140, 227–235.

Vernon, P. E. (1933). Some characteristics of the good judge of personality. *Journal of Social Psychology*, 4, 42–57.

Vorauer, J. D. and Ross, M. (1999). Self-awareness and feeling transparent: failing to suppress one's self. *Journal of Experimental Social Psychology*, 35, 415–440.

Williams, E. (2003). The relationship between momentary states of therapist self-awareness and perceptions of the counselling process. *Journal of Contemporary Psychotherapy*, 33(3), 177–186.

Williams, E. and Hill, C. (1996). The relationship between self-talk and therapy process variables for novice therapists. *Journal of Counselling Psychology*, 43, 170–177.

PART II

Self-Awareness and the Person's Experience of Illness

From health to ill health: Person experience

Assuming that people are free and autonomous (to a reasonable degree) in their own home environment, the impact of illness, depending on its severity and the resilience of individuals, can range from minor discomfort to a total sense of loss. Figure II.1 represents the impact of illness to its extreme, resulting in loss, feeling of anger, and disempowerment.

Taking on this change of role has serious implications in terms of how an individual is perceived by others. This can be explored by drawing a parallel with the notion of parenting. Obviously, parenting brings with it the added responsibility of raising children. Assuming the role of parents is natural and problem free, parents may lose the extent of their freedom and their needs become secondary to those of their children. For example, faced with the options of needing to taxi their children for swimming or music lessons and watching their favourite football team playing, it is highly improbable that parents will watch football. Interestingly, however, it is doubtful whether children are able to see their parents as human beings because all they have known is that these individuals are their mums and dads. It is not uncommon to hear such statements as *now that I have my own children, I realise what my parents must have been going through with me.* Could it be that as adults, they (the children) have developed a

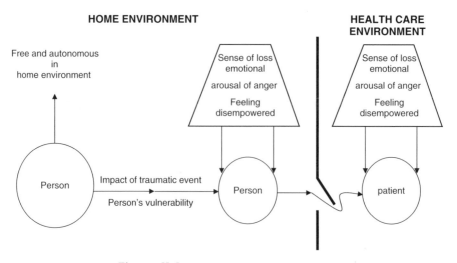

Figure II.1 Transition from person to patient.

greater sense of awareness as a result of being parents themselves? Had they not had children of their own, would they have had this awareness? Awareness of one's own role has led to parents being recognised and acknowledged as human beings. Applying a similar argument to healthy people who, arguably, through no fault of their own, have to assume the role of patients, it is not difficult to understand how the human being could be lost behind the role of patient. After all, we have always known them as patients. This begs the question, *do we wait until we too become patients before being able to realise that patients are individuals who are desperately seeking to be recognised as human beings?* The simple answer is *No.* We don't because we have at our disposal the means to recognise and acknowledge patients as people. Developing or enhancing our self-awareness is described as the best possible start to understanding others (Rungapadiachy, 1999). It could be argued that recognising the person behind the role of patient will serve to promote effective engaging. Moreover, self-awareness (as discussed in Chapter 1) holds the key to making individuals much more visible regardless of the role they occupy. Patient experience is explored through stress and vulnerability (Chapter 2), power, empowerment, and self-awareness (Chapter 3), emotion of loss and self-awareness (Chapter 4), and anger, aggression, and self-awareness (Chapter 5).

Reference

Rungapadiachy, D. M. (1999). *Interpersonal Communication and Psychology for Health Care Professionals: Theory and Practice.* Oxford: Butterworth-Heinemann.

Stress, Vulnerability, and Self-Awareness

2

Dev M. Rungapadiachy

OBJECTIVES

After reading this chapter you should be able to

▪ Discuss the notions of stress and vulnerability.

▪ Explore how stressors impact on individual vulnerability.

▪ Reflect upon how an understanding of your own vulnerability to stress can contribute to effective helping relationships.

Introduction

It could be said that although stress is a popular topic it is perhaps one of the least understood concepts in health care. The word stress is used abundantly to imply a negative force impacting on individuals, more often than not resulting in illnesses. It could also be said that some individuals would use stress as a 'get out clause' to exempt themselves from their responsibility. This last statement may come across as insensitive, however, clinical and personal experience suggests an element of truth as one colleague once said *if you tell them you are suffering from stress they become powerless and can't touch you, because even your doctor will validate your diagnosis. So you can be off sick as long as you want.* In this instance, being diagnosed as suffering from stress serves to benefit the individual. However, this is not always the case, for example stress can be a major obstacle to one's career and chances of promotion, as very few employers would want to employ someone who is vulnerable, as one employer was quoted to have said, *I don't want any deadwood in my company.* On the evidence of what has been said so far, it is not surprising to see the complex nature of stress. This chapter aims to discuss stress within the context of vulnerability in an attempt to raise one's self-awareness in relation to its effect on individuals. Self-awareness is said to give people a greater sense of control over their situation. Self-awareness is implicit within the discussion, as such no specific section is dedicated to link it with stress. However, exercises are included as a means of self-reflection. The aim is that by understanding stress from a personal perspective, one would be in a better position to engage with patients who have to endure the negative impact of stress. This chapter therefore focuses on issues related to definitions, models, vulnerability, control, and coping styles.

Defining stress

Stress has been defined as a stimulus–response (S–R) phenomenon where the stimulus makes certain demand(s) on the person who is then expected to exhibit a response of some sort. Stimulus in this instance can be called a stressor, which by definition is any agent that causes stress to an organism. Both terminologies (stress and stressor) can lead to confusion because seeing stressor as an agent of stress may imply the same thing. However, this is not the case as the term stress generally conjures up a negative connotation. The distinguishing feature of a stressor is that it has the potential to lead to a negative reaction. The point to emphasise here is that stressor may lead to stress but does not do so as a rule. For example, a married couple may go through a divorce (seen as a stressor) and only one person displays a stress reaction (negative response) in the form of depression and because the other person is not similarly affected it would be inaccurate to attribute the same meaning to both stress and stressor. An understanding of the various terminologies used in relation to stress becomes essential if one is to fully grasp the true meaning of the concept of stress. Moreover, Carpenter (1992) states that making a clear distinction between stress and stressor can account for 'wide differences in individual reactions to seemingly similar environmental demands' (p. 2). Perhaps, a more practical approach would be to view stressor as the antecedent that may or may not lead to stress depending on each individual. From Loughlin and Barling's (2000) perspective, 'stressors are the originating events or objective environmental characteristics in a given stressful situation' (p. 72). Strain is another terminology that is closely linked with stress and stressor. For example, Kessler (1983), amongst various other writers, used the terms stressor and strain interchangeably, thus implying these are one and the same thing. Strain by definition suggests an element of stretching beyond that which one is normally able to perform. Moreover, in most cases strain always leaves its mark. For example, straining a muscle would clearly suggest that an injury has taken place consequently inhibiting normal function. Strain therefore would be more accurately described as an outcome of stress. Exercise 1 emphasises your individual interpretation on the notion of stress.

EXERCISE I

Complete the following:
For me stress is . . .

In view of the fact that stress is a subjective experience therefore one could assume that it is whatever the person says stress is. For example, if I was to say that for me stress is *a feeling of being out of control and helpless in a given situation*, this means that being out of control and feeling helpless would be problematic for me to such an extent that it becomes detrimental to both my physical and mental well-being. The working definition proposed in this chapter is that of Lazarus and Launier's (1978), who argue that stress is 'any event in which environmental or internal demands (or both) *tax or exceed the adaptive resources* of an individual, social system, or tissue system' (p. 296). Individual, social, and tissue systems can be clustered under the theme of bio-psycho-social. Stress is conceptualised as a transaction between an individual and his or her environment and given that environmental demand exceeds adaptive resources the individual must mobilise more resources to maintain the status quo, and as Lazarus and Launier (1978) state, 'the more the mobilization, the greater the cost and the more likely is outcome in doubt' (p. 296).

Models of stress

There are numerous explanations as to the dynamics of a stress reaction; however, this chapter focuses predominantly on three models: Selye (1956), Holmes and Rahe (1967), and Lazarus and Folkman (1984). The origin of Selye's model could be seen to rest with Canon (1920), who saw stress as an emergency response that is commonly regarded as the 'fight or flight' response resulting from a disturbance of homeostasis under such conditions as cold, lack of oxygen, and low blood sugar (Lazarus & Folkman, 1984). Canon's idea was extended and later conceptualised by Selye (1956) as 'the general adaptation syndrome' (GAS). Whilst Selye's (1956) emphasis is principally physiological, Holmes and Rahe (1967) argue that certain environmental events require people to make changes in their established lifestyles and those who have difficulty or who are unable to readjust to these life-changing events are more likely to succumb to the negative influence stress. The main sentiment with Holmes and Rahe's model is the notion of adaptability. Lazarus and Folkman (1984) on the other hand believe that 'psychological stress is a particular relationship between the person and the environment that is appraised by the person as taxing or exceeding his or her resources and endangering his or her well-being' (p. 19). The emphasis here is that it is an individual's interpretation of his or her situation that influences the outcome of the stress dynamic.

Stress and the general adaptation syndrome

Selye (1907–1982), regarded as the founder of the stress concept (Bertók, 1998), saw stress as a set of physiological responses coordinated in such a way in order to defend against noxious agents. Selye called this organised set of bodily defences the GAS. General implies that it is produced only by agents that have a general effect upon large portions of the body. Adaptive is explained in the context of setting up defensive measures and syndrome because its individual manifestations are coordinated and even partly dependent upon each other. The basic tenet of GAS is that 'all living organisms can respond to stress as such and that, in this respect, the basic reaction pattern is always the same irrespective of the agent used to produce stress' (Selye, 1951, p. 327). According to Selye (1951), anything that causes stress endangers life unless it is met by adequate adaptive responses. Similarly, anything that endangers life causes stress and adaptive responses. Moreover, adaptability and resistance to stress are fundamental prerequisites for life and every organ and function participates in them. GAS operates at three stages, the alarm reaction, the stage of resistance, and the stage of exhaustion.

- Alarm stage is synonymous with what Selye (1982) refers to as call to arms of its defence systems. The implication is that the initial reaction to stress is shock that is followed by a counter-shock phase (Berczi, 1998). Some of the characteristic manifestations of the alarm reaction include tissue catabolism, hypoglycaemia, and gastro-intestinal erosions.

- Resistance takes place when the organism is exposed to noxious agents beyond the alarm reaction where resources are mobilised for its defence and protection. The casualty of resistance, however, is in the form of tissue damage that Selye (1956) refers to as the disease of adaptation. The manifestations present during the alarm reaction disappear during the stage of resistance.

- Exhaustion is likely to occur when there is continued resistance against the noxious agent thus resulting in a depletion of adaptive energy and the manifestations displayed during the alarm reaction reappear. Selye (1951) posits that adaptive energy is a finite quantity and its magnitude seems to 'depend largely upon genetic factors' (p. 328). The consequence of this depletion of adaptive energy can lead to death of the organism.

Stress, life events, change, and readjustment

According to Holmes and Masuda (1974), Canon's experimental work provided a necessary link in the argument that stressful life events can be harmful to health. Moreover, this link is obvious in Selye's GAS with the clear implication that death can occur as a result of depletion of adaptive energy. Research in relation to life change and illness susceptibility is seen to evolve from what is described as the chrysalis of psychobiology generated by Adolf Meyer (Holmes & Masuda, 1974). The importance of many of the life events used in Holmes and Rahe's (1967) research was, as they state, emphasised by Meyer and these include 'changes of habitat, of school entrance, graduations or changes or failures; the various jobs, the dates of possibly important births and death in the family, and other fundamentally important environmental influences' (Holmes & Rahe, 1967, p. 215). Meyer's life-charting technique, and many of the life events identified, provided for Holmes and Rahe (1967) a framework and context from which they developed the Social Readjustment Rating Scale (SRRS). The life chart device has been used systematically in over 5000 patients to study the quality and quantity of life events empirically observed to cluster at the time of disease onset. Forty-three such life events were observed under two themes and these are 'those indicative of the life style of the individual, and those indicative of occurrences involving the individual' (Holmes & Rahe, 1967, p. 216). These life-events were originally used in their laboratory to construct a schedule of recent experiences (SREs), which evolved 'mostly from ordinary social and interpersonal transactions, these events pertain to major areas of dynamic significance in the social structure of the American way of life' (Holmes & Masuda, 1967, p. 227). Life events include those that are socially desirable as well as the socially undesirable ones. Each of these life events regardless of the desirability or undesirability is linked with some coping behaviour on the part of the individual who is expected to engage in some change from his or her previous behaviour.

The participants in Holmes and Rahe's (1967) study were asked to rate each of the 43 life-changing events according to its intensity and the amount of time it would take to adjust to it. Marriage was given an arbitrary value of 500, and this served as a reference point to evaluate all other items. Participants had to ask themselves the following questions. Is this event indicative of more or less readjustment than marriage? Would the readjustment take longer or shorter to accomplish? If the chosen life event requires more readjustment than marriage a value higher than 500 is allocated. Similarly, if the life event requires less readjustment a lower value than 500 is given. And the same would apply for the time it would take to readjust. A life change unit (LCU) score was produced with death of spouse given the maximum score of 100. The score of all life events experienced was totalled to give an overall LCU score. Two further rescalings of LCU were carried out after the original study, the first in 1977 and the second in 1995. Moreover, a further 44 life events (Miller & Rahe, 1997) were added to the original study. Miller and Rahe (1997) concluded that 6-month totals equal to or greater than 300 LCU or 1-year totals equal to or greater than 500 LCU are considered indicative of high recent life stress.

Stress and cognitive appraisal

The idea of stress being described as a S–R phenomenon did not sit well with Lazarus (1993), who argues that individual differences in motivational and cognitive variables play a significant part between stimulus and response. 'All stimulus–response approaches are circular and beg the crucial questions of what it is about the stimulus that produces a particular stress response, and what it is about the response that indicates a particular stressor' (Lazarus & Folkman, 1984, p. 15). It would seem to be much more sensible to view stress as a stimulus–organism–response (S–O–R) dynamic because there are individual differences in people's vulnerability to stressors for example 'whether or not illness occurs depends on the organism's susceptibility' (Lazarus & Folkman, 1984, p. 21). The notion of vulnerability is discussed following this brief description of the cognitive appraisal model.

According to Lazarus and Folkman (1984), the judgement that a particular person–environment relationship is stressful depends very much on that person's cognitive appraisal of his or her situation. Hence, it is as the Roman philosopher Epictetus is quoted to have said that, 'people are disturbed not by things, but by the view which they take of them' (Ellis, 1989, p. 202). This would seem to provide a better explanation of individual differences in the way people respond to their particular situation. Lazarus (1990) sees stress as a transaction between an individual and his or her environment. Transaction suggests a dynamic process whereby 'stress is neither in the environmental input nor in the person, but reflects the conjunction of a person with certain motives and beliefs (personal agendas, as it were) with an environment whose characteristics pose harm, threats, or challenges depending on these person characteristics' (Lazarus, 1990, p. 3). Transaction, Lazarus (1991) argues, brings the causal variables together at a higher level of abstraction where meaning is added by the person who is confronted by the special demand from the environment. Especially significant is the concept of appraisal that underpins Lazarus and Folkman's (1984) model. This would account for individual differences in the way people react to stressful stimulus, for example an individual may respond 'with anger, another with depression, yet another with anxiety or guilt; still others feel challenged rather than threatened' (Lazarus & Folkman, 1984, p. 23). Appraisal of stressful events will determine to a large extent the nature of coping behaviour. If an individual perceives a terminal illness as a lost cause he or she may become depressed, thus passively accepting the outcome. By contrast, another person may see terminal illness as a challenge where the resulting attitude could be fight to the end. Lazarus and Folkman (1984) argue that ignoring the cognitive processes that intervene between the encounter, the reaction, and the factors that affect the nature of this mediation would inhibit our understanding of why people behave the way they do under comparable external conditions, hence the justification for cognitive appraisal as a way of explaining the concept of stress.

Cognitive appraisal is described as being much more than information processing. It is an evaluative and continuous process that occurs throughout an individual's waking life where the principal focus is on ascribing meaning to the event and establishing its relevance to self. Two types of appraisal are highlighted as primary and secondary. Lazarus and Folkman (1984) state that the choice of terminology (primary and secondary) was rather unfortunate in that primary could be construed as more important than secondary or that primary precedes secondary in time which is not the case.

Primary appraisal

Three kinds of primary appraisal – irrelevant, benign-positive, and stressful – are highlighted through evaluation of one's situation, for example faced with a stressful situation, an individual may ask, 'Am I in trouble or being benefited, now or in the future, and in what way?' (Lazarus & Folkman, 1984, p. 31).

- Irrelevance suggests that an evaluation of the situation reveals no implication for the individual. For example, there is nothing to be gained or to lose. In other words, *the situation or event does not concern me in any way.*

- Benign-positive can be seen as benefiting the individual and this is character-ised by joy, love, happiness, exhilaration, or peacefulness. There is, in most cases, always a degree of apprehension with benign-positive appraisals. For example, an individual may think, *this is too good to be true* or *this good feeling cannot last and will end in tears.*

- Stressful can be seen as harm/loss, threat, or challenge. Harm/loss suggests that some damage to the individual has already occurred such as an illness or an incapacitating injury. Threat relates to anticipated harms or losses. Lazarus and Folkman (1984) state that even when a harm/loss has occurred, it is always fused with threat because of its negative implication for the future. Challenge is described as having much in common with threat because they both demand mobilisation of coping effort. However, where challenge differs is in its potential for gain that is seen as inherent in an encounter. Challenge also generates pleasurable emotion, whereas threat is characterised by negative emotions such as fear, anxiety, and anger.

Secondary appraisal

According to Lazarus and Folkman (1984), faced with a stressful encounter whether this is a threat or a challenge people must do something to manage the situation in which they find themselves. This therefore gives rise to a different form of appraisal that they call secondary appraisal, where the focus is on *what can I do about it?* Secondary appraisal is particularly important because the outcome is contingent upon how a person responds in the face of a stressful stimulus. Moreover, this complex evaluative process 'takes into account which coping options are available, the likelihood that a given coping option will accomplish what it is supposed to and the likelihood that one can apply a particular strategy or set of strategies effectively' (Lazarus & Folkman, 1984, p. 35). For example, *what can I do about this? Will what I do serve its purpose?* Two types of expectation come into play in secondary appraisal and these are outcome expectancy and efficacy expectation. According to Bandura (1977), outcome expectancy is defined as a person's estimate that a given behaviour will lead to a certain outcome, whereas efficacy expectation is the conviction that an individual can do what it takes to overcome the problem. Secondary appraisal principally deals with coping strategies and coping skills (these are discussed later in this chapter).

Lazarus and Folkman (1984) have added a further dimension to their notion of cognitive appraisal in the form of a reappraisal that is an ongoing appraisal that takes place as a result of an individual acquiring new information relevant to their situation. The implication is that faced with a stressful event, people constantly reappraise their situation on receiving new information, thus making the initial observation in primary appraisal less stable. For example, what may have been perceived in primary appraisal as a challenge may turn out to be a threat because of doubt in one's self-efficacy.

In summary, these three models have maintained their credibility over the years principally because research support their findings. However, according to Zubin and Spring (1977), 'the main difficulty is that each model is framed so broadly that entire schools of psychopathology can pass through its portals without even rubbing shoulders' (p. 108). The implication here is that the common theme that filters through these various models is not recognised. Zubin and Spring (1977) propose the notion of vulnerability as a second-order model of stress presumably because it highlights the qualitative difference in behaviour between those who are able to adapt and those who are not able to adapt to the demand of their current or new situation. Moreover, manifestation of stress clearly rests with the individual's susceptibility. For example, Selye (1951) was clear that an individual's adaptive energy is as finite as defined by his or her genetic make-up. Moreover, Lazarus and Folkman (1984) recognise the importance of vulnerability but argue that this can be thought of as similar to the notion of potential threat 'that is transformed into active threat when that which is valued is actually put in jeopardy in a particular transaction. In this sense, vulnerability also refers to a susceptibility to react to broad classes of events with psychological stress that is shaped by a range of person factors, including commitments, beliefs, and resources' (p. 51).

The concept of vulnerability

The meaning of vulnerability is best explained though Exercise 2.

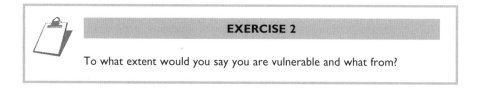

EXERCISE 2

To what extent would you say you are vulnerable and what from?

There is no doubt that most of us (if not all) are vulnerable to one thing or another at some point in our life. However, the extent of our vulnerability depends on who we are, where we are, and how we happen to behave. For example, someone who does not wear a seat belt whilst driving a motor vehicle is more vulnerable to being seriously hurt in an accident than someone who wears a seat belt. The word vulnerability is derived from the Latin verb *vulnerare* meaning to *wound*. To say that someone is vulnerable implies that he or she is in (or prone to) some sort of danger. For example, those who live near coastal areas are much more vulnerable to landslides than those who live in a city far removed from the sea (unless of course there is a big mountain in the middle of that city). Similarly, a hospital environment could be described as one that increases patients' vulnerability to infection because of Methicillin-resistant

Staphylococcus Aureus (commonly known as MRSA) or *Clostridium Difficile*. Levine (2004) states that the notion of vulnerability can be used to describe populations, individuals, their physical or psychological attributes, places, institutions, societies, and one's status in a given situation. Stress vulnerability therefore suggests that an individual is prone to suffer health problems (physical and or psychological) as a result of being exposed to stressors. The stress vulnerability model is also referred to as a diathesis-stress model (Atkinson et al., 1993). A diathesis is defined as a predisposition to a particular illness, which is developed as a consequence of stress. Zubin and Spring (1977) argue that one such illness is schizophrenia because the one thing that all sufferers have in common is 'the ever presence of their vulnerability' (p. 122). Two major types of vulnerability are identified as *inborn* and *acquired*. Inborn vulnerability is described as 'that which is laid down in the genes and reflected in the internal environment and neurophysiology of the organism', whereas acquired vulnerability is that which is the result of 'traumas, specific diseases, perinatal complications, family experiences, adolescent peer interactions, and other life events that either enhance or inhibit the development of subsequent disorder' (Zubin & Spring, 1977, p. 109). The terms diathesis and inborn vulnerability will be used interchangeably in this chapter. Exercise 3 attempts to integrate one's own vulnerability to those who have a need to access health care services.

EXERCISE 3

Imagine that you are a recipient of health care services (in- or out-patient):
How might you be vulnerable?
How would it feel to be vulnerable?
How could health care practitioners help to reduce your sense of vulnerability?

The principal aim of Exercise 3 is to raise an awareness of the notion of vulnerability as experienced by patients. The rationale is based on the principle that if I have an idea of what being vulnerable feels like for me, I can use this experience to help me understand patients' vulnerability.

Inborn vulnerability (diathesis)

In relation to psychopathology, inborn vulnerability suggests that people are generally predisposed to any given illness (Monroe & Simons, 1991). The same could be said for almost any illness, for example diabetes, heart disease, and cerebro-vascular disease (stroke). However, the onset of the illness itself depends on the extent to which people are at risk in the first place. The severity of the stressors could be seen as secondary, perhaps more as triggers than causes. Exercise 4 attempts to clarify the notion of inborn vulnerability.

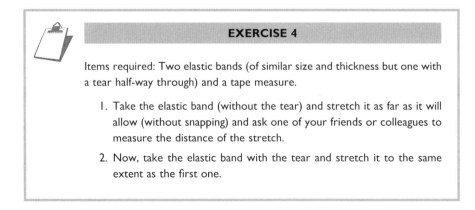

EXERCISE 4

Items required: Two elastic bands (of similar size and thickness but one with a tear half-way through) and a tape measure.

1. Take the elastic band (without the tear) and stretch it as far as it will allow (without snapping) and ask one of your friends or colleagues to measure the distance of the stretch.

2. Now, take the elastic band with the tear and stretch it to the same extent as the first one.

One can safely assume from Exercise 4 that the second elastic band snapped well before reaching the same distance as the first elastic band. Parallels can be drawn with people's vulnerability to specific illnesses, and it could be argued that those with *tear* or *weaknesses* in their genetic make-up are more susceptible to illnesses (physical and or psychological). There is no intention here to discuss the implication of genetic factors in illness vulnerability but suffice to say there is evidence to show their significance in relation to specific diseases. Other factors such as age, gender, race, and ethnicity are all implicated.

Acquired vulnerability

Acquired vulnerability is what Lazarus and Folkman (1984) see as 'person factors' in the shape of commitments and beliefs. According to Janoff-Bulman (1988), vulnerability could also be developed as a consequence of being the victim of a violent attack. The argument is based on the assumptions that prior to any serious attack, most of us hold the belief that we are *invulnerable* to such an event. Exercise 5 asks for self-reflection in relation to one's own vulnerability.

EXERCISE 5

Evaluate your own set of beliefs in relation to any event that has happened to another person. Have you ever thought that such a thing can't happen to you? Or that 'things like that only happen to irresponsible people'?

It may not be an exaggeration to say that at one time or another most of us would have held such beliefs and it is only through hindsight, direct, or indirect experience that we come to realise violent attacks can happen to anyone at anytime without being predisposed to such an event or *asking for it*. For example, we do not need to be a particular kind of person to invite violence because these can take place randomly. Janoff-Bulman (1988) states that we feel invulnerable because we hold certain core assumptions about self and the world. Three such assumptions are as follows.

- The world is benevolent that suggests not only the world is a good place to live in but its people are good as well.
- Events in the world are meaningful, simply put, we can make sense of what people do because we believe the laws of society serve to dictate and guide their behaviour.
- Self is positive and worthy in that we hold the self-belief that we are decent people who deserve respect and good treatment.

These assumptions are said to be grounded in our early preverbal experiences as children, thus their maintenance is essential to our psychological stability. However, when our assumptions are threatened we come to realise that the world is not as good a place as we thought it was, its people are not as nice as we believed them to be, and self is not inherently good but more on the lines of *there is a beast inside of everyone that is waiting to come out*. According to Janoff-Bulman (1988), becoming a victim of violence contradicts these core assumptions, hence we restructure our schema[1] to embrace the feeling of vulnerability. By contrast, people who suffer from depression hold a completely different set of assumptions that Beck (1967) calls *cognitive triad* that is characterised by holding a negative view of self, negative view of the world, and negative view of the future. According to Beck and Emery (1985), vulnerability lies at the core of anxiety disorders. The same could be said for depression. This, they argue would account for the fact that 'a particular skill that is taken for granted, and is applied smoothly and automatically under ordinary circumstances–for example, walking, talking, swimming, driving, playing an instrument–can suddenly be disturbed in the face of a threat, especially when the skill is most needed' (Beck & Emery, 1985, p. 67). Their idea of vulnerability therefore points to people's perception of themselves as subject to dangers over which they have little or no control. The ability to control is seen as a prerequisite to people's sense of safety. Moreover, the same could be said for predictability.

Controllability and predictability are the two factors that are implicit within the notion of inborn and acquired vulnerability. However, there are numerous others, for example locus of control, attributional style, learned helplessness, and types of personality that are as significant. The difficulty, however, is to cluster these according to the nature of their fit. For example, one could ask, *where does controllability fit within the context of inborn or acquired vulnerability?* One could offer a successful argument to justify its fit in either inborn or acquired vulnerability. However, it is outside the scope of this chapter to engage in such a discussion. An easy option instead is to discuss these factors in relation to the notion of vulnerability per se.

Controllability and predictability

According to Cassidy (1999), some of the factors that make a stressor stressful include its controllability and predictability. Although these are two different concepts, for the benefit of this chapter predictability is taken to be implicit within the notion of controllability. Control is defined as the belief that one has at one's disposal a response that can influence the aversiveness of an event. This implies that control does not need to be exercised for it to be effective. Moreover, it does not need to be real (as in the availability of a response that may directly influence or modify the objective characteristics of a threatening event) because perceived control may be just as effective as actual control (Thompson, 1981). In this respect, control suggests gaining mastery over one's situation by displaying coping behaviour. The coping process, however, involves reducing demand, increasing resources, or some combination of the two (Leiter, 2000). Lazarus and Folkman (1984) suggest that to cope in a given situation is to attempt to control it either by altering the environment or by managing one's own emotions and behaviour. This suggests two types of control that Rothbaum, Weizs, and Snyder (1982) call primary control, where individuals attempt to change the world so that it fits in with their individual needs, and secondary control, where individuals attempt to fit in with the needs of the world. Primary control also suggests that self is most powerful, and thus an individual is able to address the demand of the situation with reasonable ease. However, if the task itself is insurmountable individuals may readjust to fit in with the environment. Rothbaum, Weizs, and Snyder (1982) state that secondary control is likely to occur after attempts at primary control have failed. Four manifestations of secondary control are highlighted as follows.

■ **Predictive control**: If an individual comes to realise that he or she has severely limited ability to deal with demand this awareness can serve as a form of control. For example, individuals can resort to making the best of the situation thus avoid disappointment especially when they have persistently failed at some tasks. This is like finding out one's limit thus showing reasonable justification *to quit whilst ahead*.

■ **Illusory control**: This is seen as a result of attribution to chance as in luck or fate and includes belief in supernatural powers, fortune tellers, psychics, mystics, astrologers and such likes. Illusory control is indicative of perceived uncontrollability for example *it is out of my hands*. Rothbaum, Weizs, and Snyder (1982) point out that illusory control is not simply a matter of 'transformation of a perception of chance into a perception of skill. Rather, we believe that people are often aware that chance is operating and that they continue to refer to luck or fate in explaining outcomes, but that they perceive chance as a force with which they align themselves' (p. 17).

■ **Vicarious control**: This is a type of control that is apparent when an individual identifies with powerful others. For example, submitting to powerful managers or leaders enables an individual to join in their power. Vicarious control could be seen as similar to referent power (briefly explained in Chapter 3) as power based on a person's identification with or desire to be associated with the power holder. Identification is used here in a Freudian context.[2]

- **Interpretive control**: In this type of control individuals seek to understand the reasoning for the uncontrollable event in order to accept such an event. According to Rothbaum, Weizs, and Snyder (1982), 'people work hard at interpreting events so that they can accept them; in so doing, they may appear to be giving up, but their persistence suggests otherwise' (p. 24).

A distinction needs to be made here between control and perceived control. Henceforth, control will be referred to as actual control and is taken to mean *I have the potential to master the situation*. Perceived control, by contrast, is *the belief that I can master the situation in ways that leads to positive outcome*. However, the belief that one can master the situation does not make it so. For example, an individual may believe they have control over a situation but when faced with the reality of the situation discovers that demand outweighs resources. It could be argued that such realisation could have a much more negative impact on the individual. Some have suggested that perceived control could be as important as actual control (Aronson Wilson, & Akert, 1997). Also important is the role that attributions play in the S–R dynamic of stress. Attribution is the process through which people seek to explain why they do what they do. A reasonably detailed discussion regarding the notion of attribution is offered in Chapter 7. The focus here is on locus of control, attributional styles, and learned helplessness vis-à-vis vulnerability.

Locus of control

The term locus of control means *the exact position* where control of a stressor lies. According to Rotter (1966) locus of control can either be internal or external. An internal locus of control relates to the belief that one is personally responsible for what happens to oneself. Whereas an external locus of control suggests that the responsibility lies elsewhere, for example one could associate failure or success to fate, therefore *I am a victim of circumstances*. By definition therefore, an internal locus of control would offer more resistance to stress and illness. However, Cooper, Cooper, and Eaker (1988) believe that this may not necessarily be the case in some instances (for example, an individual with an internal locus of control may have even higher stress levels than someone with an external locus of control when presented with a situation over which he or she has no actual control). 'Therefore the stress relationship between locus of control and stress responses can greatly depend upon the type of stress encountered' (Cooper, Cooper, & Eaker, 1988, p. 56). Table 2.1 below gives some examples as to the types of beliefs that fall under the cluster of internal and external locus of control.

Table 2.1 Items that are considered to be internal and external locus of control

No	Internal locus of control	External locus of control
1	I am accountable for my own mistakes	Misfortunes result from bad luck
2	I get respect because I deserve it	My worth is often not recognised regardless of what I do
3	Fate or luck has nothing to do with my success	If it's meant to happen it will happen
4	For me gaining promotion depends on how hard I work	Promotion depends on being in the right place at the right time
5	What happens to me is my own doing	Life is a script and I am just an actor playing my part

Adapted from Rotter, J. B. (1966). Generalised expectancies for internal versus external control of reinforcement. *Psychological Monographs*, 80, 1–28.

Attributional styles

The motivational model of attribution, initially developed by Weiner et al. (1971), suggests that people's causal explanations for their successes or failures affect their future expectancies, affect, and behaviour. For example, if an individual performs poorly at an important task and receives negative feedback as a result, this will affect their expectations as to whether or not they can achieve success in the future. Moreover, it will affect how they feel and influence what they do in future (Martinko & Thomson, 1998). Two specific styles are highlighted as internal versus external and stable versus unstable. An internal attribution as discussed above (in internal locus of control) suggests that people perceive themselves as the cause of the outcome, such as what happens to them is of their own making. Similarly, in external attribution the outcome is seen to reside outside of the person as in the environment or with other people. The sentiment external attribution conveys is one of *Que Sera, Sera* (whatever will be will be). The stable versus unstable component relates to task difficulty or ability and whether or not the cause of the outcome changes over time. An attribution is described as stable if the person believes that his or her ability will not change and will thus never be able to succeed at a previously failed task. For example, *I failed my maths exam because I am no good with figures* and being *no good with figures* could be seen to be static and could translate to any other maths exam or any other exams that involve *figures*. Unstable attribution, on the other hand, includes effort and luck because as Martinko and Thomson (1998, p. 274) state, 'both can change over time for any specific task'. The implication is that whilst the difficulty of the task remains static, the perception of one's contribution is different because *if I work harder and with a bit of luck I could master this task*. Abramson, Seligman, and Teasdale (1978) added a further dimension to Weiner et al.'s (1971) motivation model of attributions, and 'this refers to the degree to which the cause of an outcome is generalizable across situations' (Martinko & Thomson, 1998, p. 274). The two poles of this dimension are global and specific. A global attribution is seen as perception of deficit that occurs in a broad range of situations, whereas a specific attribution relates to a narrow range

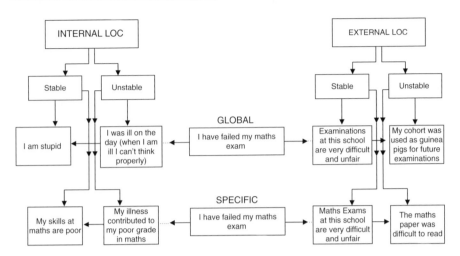

Figure 2.1   An overview of locus of control in relation to the generalisability dimension of an individual's attribution following a failed attempt at a maths examination. Based on the ideas of Abramson, L. Y., Seligman, M. E. P., and Teasdale, J. D. (1978). Learned Helpless in humans: Critique and reformulation. *Journal of Abnormal Psychology*, 87(1) 49–74.

of situations Therefore, *I am useless* would be described as global, and *I am not good with figures* would be much more specific. The dynamics between locus of control and attributional styles are summarised in Figure 2.1.

What seems to be clear is that key questions need to be asked in order to correctly identify an individual's style of attribution. For example, Weiner is quoted to have asked,

> does it apply to all the causes that we assign to behaviour? So stable–unstable is a dimension because we can sensibly ask, Is ability a factor that persists stably over time? Is patience a factor that persists stably?... Similarly, global-specific qualifies as a dimension since we can ask sensibly, Is ability a factor that affects many situations or only a few? Is patience a factor that affects many situations?
>
> (Abramson, Seligman, & Teasdale, 1978, p. 57)

From Figure 2.1, *I am stupid* is considered to be internal, stable, and global because stupidity is seen as a trait (internal) that is long-lasting (stable) and could be generalised to almost everything (global) I engage in. *I was ill on the day* is unstable because I could perform better when I am well; however, it is global since every time I am ill I may not be able to think properly hence internal (this relates to who I am). *Examinations at this school are very difficult and unfair*, seen as external, stable, and global because the school is responsible for setting examinations (external), therefore every examination that is set by the school (permanency and generalisation), not just maths examinations, is likely to be perceived as difficult and unfair. By contrast, *my skills at maths are poor* is internal, stable, and specific because skill is a personal and long-lasting characteristic but only relates to the topic maths. *Maths examinations at this school are very difficult and unfair* is described as external (outside of the individual), stable (long-lasting), and specific (relates only to maths exams).

The maths paper was difficult to read is clustered under external (the problem relates to the maths paper and not to self), unstable (paper could be made clearer), and specific (only relates to maths paper). Figure 2.1 and the explanation offered above are only meant to serve as an example of an individual's attribution styles following a failed attempt at a task and from the various permutations it can be argued that attributing failure to EXTERNAL-UNSTABLE-SPECIFIC may be far more beneficial for future behaviour than attributing failure to INTERNAL-STABLE-GLOBAL as this latter set of attribution styles contributes to learned helplessness.

Learned helplessness

Perhaps a more meaningful way to start a discussion on the topic of learned helplessness is to consider Exercise 6.

EXERCISE 6

Anticipate what your thoughts and feelings might be if you find that no matter how hard you try you just can't succeed at a given task. What impact might this have on your behaviour?

One argument suggests that repeated failure at a given task can de-motivate an individual in future trials. The concept of learned helplessness is based on similar sentiments. According to Abramson, Garber, and Seligman (1980), learned helplessness is a psychological state that frequently results when events are perceived as uncontrollable, thus resulting in a state of pessimism based on internal, stable, and global attributions. Learned helplessness was theorised to explain the behaviour of dogs that were exposed to repeated inescapable electric shocks (Seligman, 1975). As a result, these dogs seemed to give up and passively accept the painful shocks even when the experimental conditions were altered to allow them an avenue for escape. The period of inescapable shocks seemed to have *sapped* the dogs' energy and motivation, rendering them unable to avoid future shocks. According to Seligman (1975), 'when an organism has experienced trauma it cannot control, its motivation to respond in the face of later trauma wanes' (p. 22). Numerous experiments have been conducted using human subjects who were placed in uncontrollable situations, and the results were similar to those found with dogs (see Hiroto, 1974). The learned helplessness theory hypothesises that 'learning that outcomes are uncontrollable results in three deficits: motivational, cognitive, and emotional' (Abramson, Seligman, & Teasdale, 1978, p. 50). Motivational deficit is taken to mean the retarded initiation of voluntary responses as a consequence of the expectation that outcomes are uncontrollable. For example, if people come to expect that their action is futile and will in no way influence the outcome, the likelihood is that most of them would stop trying. However, exposure to an uncontrollable event itself would not be sufficient to lead to cognitive deficit. The organism must come to expect that the outcome is beyond its control. In relation to emotional deficit, Abramson, Seligman, and Teasdale (1978) posit that depression results upon learning that one's action is independent of outcomes.

There are two types of helplessness and these are universal and personal. Universal helplessness is said to result when people come to believe that neither they nor anyone else can solve their problem. A terminal illness such as some types of leukaemia would be a typical example where people may feel neither they nor anyone else can help possibly because as yet there may be no known cure. Personal helplessness, on the other hand, is said to be present when individuals come to believe that outcome is non-contingent on their response. For example, no matter how hard I try I can't figure out a solution to my problem. This, however, does not mean that the problem is unsolvable as others may be able to solve it on their behalf.

Peterson and Seligman (1987) propose six pathways that serve as possible links between attributional style and physical well-being. People who hold internal, stable, and global explanations are vulnerable to the following behaviour.

- They may become passive following an illness by not seeking or following medical advice and are thus more likely to exacerbate their illness.

- They may neglect the basics of health care in the first instance because they might not see the link between their behaviour and their illness.

- They tend not to be good problem solvers when faced with uncontrollability. This therefore leads to a vicious cycle where inability to address one problem leads to more problems.

- They tend to be socially withdrawn and are thus deprived of social contacts with others that could have acted as a buffer to illness.

- They may suffer depression and are thus at greater risk of physical illnesses.

- They may have less competent immune systems resulting from their sense of uncontrollability of an event.

From what has been said thus far it becomes clear that personal factors are significant to one's resistance to the negative effects of stress. Two such factors that form part of the ensuing discussion are Friedman and Rosenman's (1974) type A and B behaviour patterns and Kobassa's (1979) concept of hardiness.

Type A and type B behaviour pattern

According to Friedman and Rosenman (1974), type A behaviour pattern (TABP) is described as 'an action–emotion complex that can be observed in any person who is aggressively involved in a chronic, incessant struggle to achieve more and more in less and less time, and if required to do so, against the opposing efforts of other things or person' (p. 67). By contrast, type B behaviour pattern (TBBP) is the absence of type A behaviour. According to Van Egeren (1991) TABP reflects current cultural attitudes in that 'the fierce competitiveness, the preoccupation with success, the staking of self-worth on success, the inner tyranny of unreasonable expectations of self and others – are common in our society' (p. 45). Van Egeren (1991) argues that despite this uncompromising drive to succeed, type A people usually end up failing to gain those things that matter most in life such as, happiness, self-acceptance, and peace of mind. Moreover, TABP is implicated as a risk factor for coronary heart disease. According to Glass (1977), some of the descriptive characteristics of TABP include the following.

- **Striving for competitive achievement**: TABP shows an intense drive to succeed in achievement-related activities. For example, these individuals would work at their near maximum capacity even in the absence of a specific deadline for task completion. However, they tend to suppress feelings of fatigue in the process to a greater extent than TBBP.

- **Exaggerated sense of time urgency**: TABP has a tendency to do more in less time. Moreover, Glass (1977) found that individuals with the A traits show greater impatience and irritation when delayed in the execution of their activities than individuals with B traits.

- **Aggressiveness and hostility**: Hostility and aggression are not easily detected in type A individuals as they 'often keep such affect and reactions under cover' (Glass, 1977, p. 66). However, there is sufficient evidence to support the notion that individuals with type A disposition are more likely to show aggressiveness and hostility than type B individuals.

The characteristics displayed by type A seem to suggest that these individuals are more vulnerable to illness than type B. One of the key contributory factors indicates that type A individuals have a desperate need to control their environment. Moreover, when these individuals feel that control is slipping away from them, they experience a great deal of stress that could have a negative impact on their health. However, according to Phares and Chaplin (1997), there are several personality characteristics that appear to serve as a stress buffer. One such factor is the hardiness of personality.

Hardiness of personality

Kobasa (1979) proposes that people who experience high degrees of stress without falling ill have a personality structure, characterised by the term hardiness that differentiates them from people who become sick under stress. Kobasa (1979) argues that individuals who are hardy possess three general characteristics.

1. **The belief that they can control or influence the events of their experience**: This sense of self-efficacy serves to influence health status positively. For example, hardy individuals are more likely to structure their life with a clear sense of their values, goals, and capabilities, and a belief in their importance. Hence, they show commitment instead of alienation from self.

2. **The ability to feel deeply involved in or committed to activities of their lives**: These individuals would take a very active part in their lives thus immersing themselves in more or less everything they engage in.

3. **The anticipation of change is regarded as an exciting challenge to personal development**: Here change is perceived to be meaningful in that it 'can be transformed into a potential step in the right direction' in one's life (Kobasa, 1979, p. 9).

Some researches support the idea that hardiness contributes to the avoidance of illness. For example, Roth et al. (1989) argue that their study provides ample opportunity to demonstrate the stress-buffering effects of hardiness and fitness. The implication is that both hardiness and fitness are associated with health in general. They do add, however, that when unique or independent predictive effects were examined only fitness remained clearly related to health. For Funk and Houston (1987), interesting though the concept of hardiness may be, it has significant shortcomings [see Funk and Houston (1987) for a detailed discussion].

Stress and coping styles

It is generally acknowledged that people are continuously exposed to stressful life events. However, their ability (perceived or real) to deal with these stressors is likely to dictate whether or not they suffer the negative impact of stress. It can be safely assumed that if individuals can readjust to new demands of the environment, they will experience little or no stress. One could deduce from this that coping styles are more significant in determining the outcome of a stressful life event than the event itself. Exercise 7 encourages you to explore your own coping mechanisms.

EXERCISE 7

Faced with what you consider to be a stressful life event (work with an example), explain how you may behave? You may use previous experience to guide your answer.

Reflecting on Lazarus and Folkman's (1984) model of stress, coping strategies are linked with the notion of secondary appraisal where individuals establish whether or not they can cope with the demand of their environment. According to Sideridis (2006), this represents action tendencies to alter the person–environment relationship by resourcing cognitive and behavioural energies to enable the person to cope with the demand of the environment. However, Folkman and Lazarus (1985) state that the essence of stress, coping, and adaptation rest with the notion of change where both emotion and coping are implicated. Neither emotion nor coping are static, for example, 'at first one may feel anxious; after a few moments of further interchange, angry; then guilt; then loving and joyful. The sequence of feelings reflects the changing meaning or significance of what is happening as the encounter unfolds' (Folkman & Lazarus, 1985, p. 150). Moreover, behaviourally 'one might at first engage in avoidant or denial-like strategies to ward off the significance of an event, then decide to deal head-on with the problem; or at the stressful outset a person might cope by avoiding contact with others but a little later seek emotional support from a friend' (Folkman & Lazarus, 1985, p. 150). Emotions are seen to have a diagnostic value in that they can reveal how people think they are managing. Coping is referred to as both cognitive and behavioural efforts to manage what Folkman and Lazarus (1985) call 'a troubled person–environment relationship' (p. 152). Two types of coping are highlighted as emotion and problem focused. Emotion-focused coping suggests that energy is spent on regulating the distressing emotions associated with problems that one may encounter. In problem-focused coping energy is spent by addressing the actual problem.

Reflecting on Exercise 7 and in relation to emotion and problem-focused coping, you might like to identify which coping style you would have adopted. Whether individuals adopt an emotion or a problem-focused approach to manage their problem is perhaps less important than the consequence of that approach. Moreover, Lazarus (1999) believes that coping must be measured separately from its outcomes in order to determine the effectiveness of each coping strategy. It would be erroneous therefore to suggest one approach is superior to another. However, Austenfeld and Stanton (2004) believe that emotion-focused coping has earned itself a 'bad reputation' in coping literature by being associated with dysfunctional outcomes (maladaptive), whereas problem-focused coping is perceived as a more adaptive strategy. Lazarus (1999) is clear that this is far from the truth and argues that in fact both emotion and problem-focused coping styles can co-exist. Lazarus (1999, p. 123) states,

> if a person takes a Diazepam pill before an exam because of distressing and disabling test anxiety, a little thought will show that this act serves both functions, not just one. Although the emotion and its physiological sequels, such as excessive arousal, dry mouth, trembling, and intrusive thoughts about failing, will be reduced, performance is also improved because these symptoms will now interfere less with the performance. The coper's intentions are often consciously to achieve both goals. We should have learned by now that the same act may have more than one function and usually does.

It could be said therefore that both emotion and problem-focused coping styles are useful in their own rights. For example, Lazarus (1984) found that when conditions of stress are perceived to be within one's control then problem-focused coping was more apparent. Moreover, when conditions of stress are appraised to be beyond one's control then emotion-focused coping predominates. It could be argued therefore that a coping style can only be classed as maladaptive if and when it exacerbates the problem.

Summary

Stress is a complex phenomenon where individual interpretation of events seems to influence its impact on the person. However, impact is dictated by one's vulnerability that is seen as inborn and/or acquired. Inborn vulnerability suggests being predisposed to stressful life events, for example illnesses with a genetic basis. Acquired vulnerability points to person factors that are embedded in individuals' commitments and beliefs. Learning also plays an important role in that it can serve, as a foundation for future behaviour such is the case with learned helplessness. The principal element underpinning learned helplessness is the notion of controllability. Learned helplessness is said to occur when an organism is not able to influence the outcome of an event. However, attribution and coping styles are two significant factors in the stress–environment dynamics. Internal, stable, and global attributions are more likely to result in learned helplessness. Emotion and problem-focused coping styles are two strategies employed in dealing with stressful life events. Moreover, equal emphasis should be placed on both emotion and problem-focused coping because these are found to be dictated by the nature of the stressful event.

References

Abramson, L. Y., Garber, J., and Seligman, M. E. P. (1980). Learned helplessness in humans: an attributional analysis. In Garber, J. and M. E. P. Seligman (eds.), *Human Helplessness: Theory and Applications* (pp. 3–34). New York, London, Toronto, Sydney, and San Francisco: Academic Press.

Abramson, L. Y., Seligman, M. E. P., and Teasdale, J. (1978). Learned helpless in humans: critique and reformulation. *Journal of Abnormal Psychology*, 87, 49–74.

Aronson, E., Wilson, T. D., and Akert, R. M. (1997). *Social Psychology*. New York: Longman.

Atkinson, R. L., Atkinson, R. C., Smith, E. E., and Bem, D. J. (1993). *Introduction to Psychology*. New York, Toronto, Montreal, London, Sydney, and Tokyo: Harcourt, Brace, and Company.

Austenfeld, J. L. and Stanton, A. L. (2004). Coping through emotional approach: a new look at emotion, coping, and health-related outcomes. *Journal of Personality*, 72(6), 1335–1363.

Bandura, A. (1977). Self-efficacy: toward a unifying theory of behavioural change. *Psychological Review*, 84(2), 191–215.

Beck, A. T. (1967). *Depression: Clinical, Experimental, and Theoretical Aspects*. New York: Harper & Row. Republished as *Depression: Causes and Treatment*. Philadelphia: University of Pennsylvania Press, 1972.

Beck, A. T. and Emery, G. (1985). *Anxiety Disorders and Phobias: a Cognitive Perspective*. New York: Basic Books.

Berczi, I. (1998). The stress concept and neuroimmunoregulation in modern biology. In P. Csermely (ed.), *Stress of Life: From Molecules to Man* (pp. 3–12). New York: The New York Academy of Science.

Bertók, L. (1998). Stress and non-specific resistance. In P. Csermely (ed.), *Stress of Life: From Molecules to Man* (pp. 1–2). New York: The New York Academy of Science.

Canon, W. (1920). *Bodily Changes in Pain, Hunger, Fear and Rage: An Account of Recent Researches into the Function of Emotional Excitement*. New York and London: Appleton and Company.

Carpenter, B. (1992). Issues and advances in coping research. In B. Carpenter (ed.), *Personal Coping: Theory, Research, and Application* (pp. 1–13). Westport: Praeger.

Cassidy, T. (1999). *Stress, Cognition and Health*. London: Routledge.

Cooper, C. L., Cooper, R. D., and Eaker, L. H. (1988). *Living with Stress*. London: Penguin Books.

Ellis, A. (1989). Rational-emotive therapy. In R. J. Corsini and D. Wedding (eds.), *Current Psychotherapies*. Itasca: F. E. Peacock Publishers, Inc.

Folkman, S. and Lazarus, R. (1985). If it changes, it must be a process. Study of emotion and coping during three stages of a college examination. *Journal of Personality and Social Psychology*, 48, 150–170.

Friedman, M. and Rosenman, R. H. (1974). *Type A Behaviour and Your Heart*. New York: Knopf.

Funk, S. C. and Houston, B. K. (1987). A critical analysis of the hardiness scale's validity and utility. *Journal of Personality and Social Psychology*, 53(3), 572–578.

Glass, D. C. (1977). *Behaviour Patterns, Stress, and Coronary Disease*. Hillsdale, NJ: Lawrence Erlbaum Associates, Inc.

Hiroto, D. S. (1974). Locus of control and learned helplessness. *Journal of Experimental Psychology*, 102, 187–193.

Holmes, T. H. and Masuda, M. (1974). Life changes and illness susceptibility. In B. S. Dohrenwend and B. P. Dohrenwend (eds.), *Stressful life events: Their Nature and Effects* (pp. 45–72). New York: John Wiley and Sons.

Holmes, T. H. and Rahe, R. H. (1967). The social readjustment scale. *Journal of Psychosomatic Research*, 11, 213–218.

Janoff-Bulman, R. (1988). Victims of violence. In S. Fisher and J. Reason (eds.), *Handbook of Life Stress, Cognition and Health* (pp. 101–113). Chichester and New York: John Wiley and Sons.

Kessler, R. C. (1983). Methodological issues in the study of psychosocial stress. In H. B. Kaplan (ed.), *Psychosocial Stress: Trends in Theory and Research* (pp. 267–341). New York and London: Academic Press.

Kobassa, S. C. (1979). Stressful life events, personality and health: an inquiry into hardiness. *Journal of Personality and Social Psychology*, 37, 1–11.

Lazarus, R. S. (1984). On the primacy of cognition. *American Psychologist*, 39, 124–129.

Lazarus, R. S. (1990). Theory-based measurement. *Psychological Inquiry*, 1(1), 3–13.

Lazarus, R. S. (1991). Cognition and motivation. *American Psychologist*, 46(4), 352–367.

Lazarus, R. S. (1993). Coping theory and research: past, present, and future. *Psychosomatic Medicine*, 55, 234–247.

Lazarus, R. S. (1999). *Stress and Emotion: A New Synthesis*. London: Free Association Books.

Lazarus, R. S. and Folkman, S. (1984). *Stress, Appraisal, and Coping*. New York: Springer Publishing Company.

Lazarus, R. and Launier, R. (1978). Stress-related transaction between and environment. In L. A. Pervin and M. Lewis (eds.), *Perspectives in Interactional Psychology* (pp. 189–187). New York and London: Plenum press.

Leiter, T. (2000). Organizational change: adaptive coping and the need for training. In P. Dewe, M. Leiter, and T. Cox (eds.), *Coping, Health and Organizations* (pp. 125–143). London and New York: Taylor and Francis.

Levine, C. (2004). The concept of vulnerability in disaster research. *Journal of Traumatic Stress*, 17(5), 395–402.

Loughlin, C. and Barling, J. (2000). Coping with acute workplace disasters. In P. Dewe, M. Leiter, and T. Cox (eds.), *Coping, Health and Organizations* (pp. 71–85). Boca Raton, London, New York, and Washington, DC: CRC Press.

Martinko, M. J. and Thomson, N. F. (1998). A synthesis and extension of the weiner and kelly attribution models. *Basic and Applied Social Psychology*, 20(4), 271–284.

Miller, M. A. and Rahe, R. H. (1997). Life changes scaling for the 1990s. *Journal of Psychosomatic Research*, 43(3), 279–292.

Monroe, S. M. and Simons, A. D. (1991). Diathesis-stress theories in the context of life-stress research: implications for the depressive disorders. *Psychological Bulletin*, 110, 406–425.

Peterson, C. and Seligman, M. E. P. (1987). Explanatory style and illness. *Journal of Personality*, 55(2), 237–265.

Phares, E. J. and Chaplin, W. F. (1997). *Introduction to Personality*. New York and Harlow: Longman.

Roth, D. L., Wiebe, D. J., Fillingim, R. B., and Shay, K. A. (1989). Life events, fitness, hardiness, and health: a simultaneous analysis of proposed stress-resistance effects. *Journal of Personality and Social Psychology*, 57(1), 136–142.

Rothbaum, F., Weizs, J. R. and Snyder, S. S. (1982). Changing the world and changing self: a two process model of perceived control. *Journal of Personality and Social Psychology*, 42, 5–37.

Rotter, J. B. (1966). Generalised expectancies for internal versus external control of reinforcement. *Psychological Monographs*, 80, 1–28.

Seligman, M. E. P. (1975). *Helplessness*. San Francisco: W. H. Freeman.

Selye, H. (1951). The general adaptation syndrome. *Annual Review of Medicine*, 2, 327–342.

Selye, H. (1956). *The Stress of Life*. New York: McGraw-Hill Book Company.

Selye, H. (1982). History and present status of the stress concept. In L. Goldberger and S. Breznitz (eds.), *Handbook of Stress: Theoretical and Clinical Aspects* (pp. 7–17). New York: Free Press.

Sideridis, G. D. (2006). Coping is not an 'either' 'or': the interaction of coping strategies in regulating affect arousal and performance. *Stress and Health*, 22, 315–327.

Thompson, S. C. (1981). Will it hurt less if I can control it? A complex answer to a simple question. *Psychological Bulletin*, 90, 89–101.

Van Egeren, L. (1991). A 'success trap' theory of type a behaviour: historical background. In M. J. Strube (ed.), *Type A Behaviour* (pp. 45–58). Newbury Park, London, and New Delhi: Sage Publications.

Weiner, B., Frieze, I., Kukla, A., Reed, L. Rest, S., and Rosenbaum, R. M. (1971). *Perceiving the Causes of Success and Failure*. Morristown, NJ: General Learning Press.

Zubin, J. and Spring, B. (1977). Vulnerability: a new view of schizophrenia. *Journal of Abnormal Psychology*, 86(2), 103–126.

Power, Empowerment, and Self-Awareness in Helping Relationships

Steve Howarth and Dev M. Rungapadiachy

OBJECTIVES

After reading this chapter you should be able to

▪ Demonstrate an understanding of the concept of power in relation to self and others.

▪ Discuss the impact of power in helping relationships.

▪ Reflect upon ways of empowering patients through effective engagement.

Introduction

Power in the context of health service delivery seems to be implicitly attributed to health care professionals in particular doctors as having the upper hand in their relationship with patients. 'Disempowerment' on the other hand is attributed to those who access health care services with the implication that they are disadvantaged by virtue of their sick role. The origin of the term sick role can be traced back to Parsons (1951), who sees the sick as failing in some way to fulfil one or more of their roles in society. Illness is seen as a state of affairs that impairs, in varying ways and degrees, the capacity of the sick person to function. For Parsons (1975), 'the privilege of exemption from ordinary day-to-day occupations which has gone with the institutionalization of the sick role is a kind of institutional measure of incapacity when it is combined with the fundamental tenet that being ill, if it is genuine and not malingering, cannot reasonably be regarded as the sick person's "fault" ' (p. 259). However, there was generally a belief that patients were motivated to remain sick through resisting therapeutic efforts on the part of health care professionals, perceived as agents of social control. Doctors, in particular, by virtue of their 'expert' role were regarded as important in maintaining individuals' social responsibilities. It could be argued that under the expert model of care, the distribution of power between health care professionals and service users is perceived to be in favour of the former. Goffman (1961) argues that whenever there is an imbalance of power between two parties the least powerful becomes the most vulnerable and at risk party, as was evident at Alder Hey hospital (Hunter, 2001) and currently at Guantanamo Bay.[1] Contemporary approaches to health service delivery see an attempt to move away from the expert model by embracing the concept of patient empowerment through client-centred care (Rogers, 1946) and a patient-led NHS (DoH, 2005a). The implication is that patients will have greater control and 'a far greater range of choices and of information and help to make choices' (DoH, 2005a, p. 5). As a response to events at Alder Hey, the then Health Secretary, Alan Milburn stated that the relationship between patients and the service today has to be based on informed consent. One of The British Government's objectives is to increase patients' power by shifting the balance of power within the NHS. For example, 'we need to develop a patient centred service where patients are seen as active partners in their care' (DoH, 2001, p. 12). Moreover, 'patients and the public will be more involved in the NHS, as the NHS moves towards a model of increased partnership, with patients and the public having their say in how services are designed, developed and delivered' (DoH, 2001, p. 6). However, as Canter (2001) argues, shifting power in favour of the patient may not be so straightforward, possibly, because of the notion that power is much more complex than it appears. This chapter therefore explores the concepts of power and disempowerment in the context of a helping relationship through self-awareness.

The concept of power

A starting point to understand power is with Exercise 1.

EXERCISE 1

Make a list of all the words that come to mind when you think of power. Whilst exploring your list, deduce a common sentiment or common sentiments that these words convey to you.
From what you have deduced, define what power means to you.

The words that emerged as a result of a brainstorming session with one of our student groups are found in Appendix 1. On closer examination it can be deduced that the common theme seems to point towards an intrinsic energy force (physical and/or psychological) that *may* be used to influence someone. The stress is on may because it does not necessarily follow that people who have power use it all the time. Dowding (1996) clarifies this by defining power as a dispositional concept, for example, as lecturers we have the power to refuse students entry to lectures if they arrive late (but I would not exercise this power). Power as a dispositional concept is reflected in Weber's (1947) definition, that is 'the probability that one actor within a social relationship will be in a position to carry out his own will despite resistance' (p. 152). Dowding (1996) also sees power as a two-dimensional concept, 'power to' and 'power over' (p. 4). *Power to* is taken to mean having the ability to perform an act, whatever this act may be. However, when the act involves getting someone to do something, for example, students to present seminars as a module requisite, the term *power over* would seem to be more appropriate. *Power to* and *power over* are referred to as outcome power and social power, respectively (Dowding, 1996). This chapter focuses predominantly on social power.

A classic definition of social power is the capacity of some persons to produce intended and foreseen effects on others (Wrong, 1979). In recognising the problematic nature of this definition, Wrong (1979) describes some key issues that would need to be considered for a fuller understanding of the meaning of power. The issues discussed here are intentionality, effectiveness, latent or potential, and asymmetry.

Intentionality

Generally speaking, the intention to influence another person seems to be inherent within the dynamic of power. However, direct power or its symbolic representations can also influence people unintentionally. For example, we may drive our car with some anxieties while trying hard to keep to the speed limit when followed by a police patrol car. It could be argued therefore that it is not police officers' intention to cause anxiety but instead the inherent power by virtue of their role. 'The effects others have on us, unintended by and even unknown to them, may influence us more profoundly and permanently than direct efforts to control our sentiments and behaviour' (Wrong, 1979, p. 4). This unintended influence can be regarded as one of the most fundamental issues within any interaction that involves health care practitioners and patients. Exercise 2 offers a structure to enhance awareness of the unintended effect that your role may have on another individual.

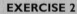

EXERCISE 2

In your personal or professional role, identify one individual who is subordinate to you.
Wherever possible discuss with him or her the unintended effect your behaviour may have on this person.

As health professionals it is essential that we attempt to understand the unintended effect we may have on those that we interact with, be they health care students or patients.

Effectiveness

One could argue that the exercise of power can be both effective or ineffective (successful or unsuccessful) depending on the outcome of our influence. However, one can only say one has power when one's attempt to influence others is successful and the desired outcome is achieved. Power therefore can only be perceived through successful influence of others.

Latent or potential power

This type of power refers to one's ability to control or influence others even in one's absence. For example, a consultant physician may have given orders not to resuscitate a patient who is terminally ill. This order will most likely be carried out even in the physician's absence. In such instances, the physician would be said to have latent or potential power. Some would say that power is always potential (Bierstedt, 1974). However, it could be argued that this is not always the case, for example, it is also possible that *while the cat is away, the mouse will play*. Here, although we are aware of our superiors' orders we may not necessarily *toe the line* in their absence unless of course *big brother* is watching in which case it would not be seen as latent power.

Asymmetry and balance of power

Power by definition suggests an asymmetrical relationship between the power holder and the power object. For example, there can never be symmetry between parents and children, employers and employees, teachers and students, and health care professionals and patients. According to Wrong (1979), it would be contradictory to refer to a relationship between two parties as having equal power. Moreover, Blau (1964) states that the source of power 'is one-sided dependence. Interdependence and mutual influence of equal strength indicate lack of power' (p. 118). Consider the question in Exercise 3.

EXERCISE 3

If Blau's statement is true, how feasible do you think the government's objective of shifting the balance of power from health care professionals to that of patients is?

In any relationship, if service providers have something that we desperately need this automatically places us in a subservient position, power then would be clearly situated with them unless of course we are able to satisfy our needs elsewhere. It could be said therefore that the true essence of power is asymmetrically based. In examining the concept of power dependence, Blau (1967) posits four options that are available to anyone who needs a service that someone else has to offer.

- We can get the service provided we have the resources to do so. For example, at a time when crisis is looming in the provision of dental care in the United Kingdom we can still obtain care as long as we are prepared to opt for private treatment. This, however, would involve reciprocal exchanges, and power still rests with the service provider.

- We can try and obtain the service elsewhere if it is available. In this instance we may be seen to have bargaining power.

- We can coerce a service provider, if we are able to do so, to offer us the service. Power in this case would be seen to rest with us.

- We may learn to resign ourselves to do without this service. Here, we would be perceived as powerless.

It could be argued that if power is shifted from health care professionals to patients then this must mean that patients should be able to influence health care professionals. However, it is questionable whether health care professionals, as a whole, are ready and willing for such a transformation. One can only reiterate that power in any event can only be perceived as an asymmetrical concept where one person (the power holder) is in a position to influence another (the power object).

Power through

According to Turner (2005), a further dimension needs to be explored in order to fully understand power. The concept of *power through* as Turner (2005) calls it suggests 'the capacity to affect the world, including others, through influencing and controlling people to carry out one's will, to act on one's behalf, as an extension of oneself' (p. 6). The two emerging sub-categories of *power through* are influence and control.

Power through influence (persuasion)

Most of what has been offered thus far emphasises power through influence and implies our ability to persuade others that what we would like them to do is right and just. Turner (2005) posits that, 'if one can persuade others of the correctness of some belief or the rightness of some action, then they are likely to act on it as a matter of their own volition, as free, intrinsically motivated and willing agents' (pp. 6–8).

Power through control

Power through control is different to power through influence in that when it is used in the former sense, the subject of one's power does not have to be persuaded or even interested in the 'right and wrong' of the act to be performed.

According to Turner (2005), power through control is the 'capacity to get people to do what one wants where they are *not* persuaded of or are *uninterested* in the validity of the specific act' (p. 8). This sounds more like having no choice but to carry out an act as ordered, for example, we do not have the free will to disobey. Control can be exercised through legitimate authority and coercion. Control through legitimate authority suggests that power holders, by virtue of their positions within the group structure, own the right to get the power object to do as they prescribe. This is seen as legitimate power. For example, when asked to stop by a police officer one has little choice but to obey. Here it could be argued that people have been socialised into accepting the role of the power holder. As Turner (2005) states, 'control is based on voluntary deference to and private acceptance of ingroup authority' (p. 8). Control can also take place through coercion where people are controlled against their wishes. For example, people may be denied a life-saving treatment if they continue to smoke cigarettes. The implication is that people are forced to act according to the will of the power holder, and in the process they act against their own will. This sentiment is reflected in the concept of obedience, which forms part of a later discussion. According to French and Raven (1959), legitimate power and coercive power are two of the five sources of power. The remaining three sources are reward power, referent power, and expert power. Reward power suggests that the power holder is perceived as having the ability to bring about a positive outcome. Referent power is based on a person's identification with or desire to be associated with the power holder. For example, if we like the power holder we are more likely to be readily influence by him or her. Expert power is indicated when we perceive a person to be able to provide us with special knowledge. For example, patients would perceive health care professionals as experts in health matters. Legitimate and coercive power will most likely lead to obedience, whereas reward, referent, and expert power may lead to compliance and conformity.

Obedience

Obedience can be seen as the most direct form of social influence that involves orders typically from an acknowledged authority figure where people feel compelled to obey direct orders. According to Milgram (1974), 'the person who, with inner conviction, loathes stealing, killing, and assault may find himself performing these acts with relative ease when commanded by authority' (p. xi). Milgram's statement clearly demonstrates his strong belief about the power of authority. In an attempt to find out how many people would resist orders (immoral requests) from authority figures, Milgram (1963)[2] conducted a series of experiments where his participants were led to believe that they were taking part in an investigation to study the effects of punishment on learning. The nature of one particular experiment required two participants, a learner and a teacher. The selection of learner and teacher was made to appear as if these were randomly allocated when in fact the learner was a confederate[3] and the teacher was the unknowing subject. In this particular experiment both the learner and the teacher were taken to a room where the learner was strapped to a chair, with electrodes attached to his arms. The learner was told that a list of simple word pairs will be read to him and he will then be tested on his ability to remember the second word of a pair. For example, the word pair was read to the learner once, then the teacher would read the first word of each pair followed by four possible answers. The learner would press a button to indicate his response. The learner is also informed that he will receive electric shocks whenever he makes a mistake. Moreover, each shock will increase in intensity. For example, if the learner makes a mistake at word pair one he receives 15 volts, at word pair two, 30 volts, and so on. The teacher was then taken to an adjacent room with a 'shock generator' that had 30 switches. The experimenter explained that the switch on the far left administers a very mild (15 volts) shock and each succeeding switch increases the shock by 15 volts. Switch number 30 on the far right delivers 450 volts. The switches are also labelled from left to right as 'slight shock, moderate shock, very strong shock', and at the far right, 'danger-severe shock'. The last two switches on the far right were labelled 'XXX'. The teacher was given a sample shock of 45 volts prior to the start of the experiment to create a more realistic impression of the experiment as the 'jolt strengthened the subjects's belief in the authenticity of the machine' (Milgram, 1974, p. 20). However, the learner never received any shock.

Milgram himself could not have predicted what he found. In fact, prior to the experiment, he surveyed a number of people from various walks of life, psychiatrists, college students, and middle class adults, and almost all predicted that the subjects would refuse to obey. Psychiatrists in particular, said that most subjects would not go beyond 150 volts. However, the result of the first experiment shows that out of 40 participants (teacher role) who took part 25 obeyed the orders to carry on until the end of the experiment. This meant that the victim (learner) was punished until the most potent shock on the generator was reached. This particular experiment shows over 65% of the participants were fully obedient. However, according to Milgram (1974), similar experiments were carried out in Munich, Rome, South Africa, and Australia, and the level of obedience was reported to be higher than that found in the first experiment. Moreover, the experiment in Munich revealed an 85% level of obedience. Milgram (1974) posits that the essence of obedience is that people come to view themselves as the instrument for carrying out other people's wishes. Therefore, they no longer regard themselves as responsible for their actions. The most far-reaching consequence of this shift of attitude is that people feel responsible to the authority directing them, but they do not feel responsible for the content of the actions that the authority prescribes. 'Morality does not disappear but acquires a radically different focus: the subordinate person feels shame or pride depending on how adequately he has performed the actions called for by authority' (Milgram, 1974, p. 146). Exercise 4 encourages self-reflection in relation to being the instrument of power.

As a student of health care one may feel a sense of comfort to know that the responsibility lies with the qualified staff. However, one's duty of care would need to be taken into account.

EXERCISE 4

Reflect on one or two occasions when you did not see yourself as responsible for your action, the responsibility instead was with the person who gave the orders. How does it feel to know that someone else is responsible for what you do?

What can we learn from Milgram's (1974) experiment on obedience? One of the principal messages is that one should never underestimate the nature of the social situation because the power of influence works in ways beyond one's expectation. We know that some of Milgram's subjects inflicted maximum shock to the learners not because they were sadistic. Quite the contrary, because when the subjects were under orders but free to choose the level of shock they can administer this only averaged at below 60 volts. The implication is that the reason for obedience clearly rests with how they perceived authority. In most cases authority was perceived as *it's my duty to carry out orders,* and this resulted in shifting responsibility to the authority figure, and in doing so the subjects felt morally exonerated from the act. Milgram's experiments could be seen as dated; however, personal experience suggests that obedience and to some extent blind obedience is rife within health care system. Patients tend to blindly obey health care professionals who in turn obey their superiors. This begs the question, why do we obey? Exercise 5 encourages you to reflect obedience in relation to self and patients.

EXERCISE 5

Reflect on your own place of work and identify whom do your patients obey and why? Similarly whom do you yourself obey and why?

It could be said that one of the principal reasons for obedience is the way we are socialised from the time we are little children. We are brought up to obey and respect our parents, elders, teachers, doctors, and people in authority. There is generally an expectation for people to obey and those who do not are perceived as deviant.

Lack of social comparison is also a possible reason for people's obedience. For example, when individuals are on their own, they do not have the opportunity to compare their ideas and feelings with others. These individuals have no idea what others would do in a similar situation. The presence of others therefore is significant in terms of whether a person disobeys (Milgram, 1965). This is often reflected in classroom behaviour. For example, when students are asked to take part in an activity of say, 'self-presentation' that involves talking about themselves, very often as soon as one person says he or she can't think of what to say others would follow suit. It is as if precedence has been set and others tend to use this as a template for future behaviour. Chances are if people don't have this precedence they will most likely obey.

Perception of legitimate authority is another significant factor for obedience; however, it is not fully responsible for it. For example, when Milgram (1974) replicated his study in a different setting to that of Yale University, obedience dropped from 65% to 48%. The drop in obedience rate is attributed to the prestige that Yale University commands.

Obedience is also enhanced by what could be called 'foot-in-the-door technique' (see Gilbert, 1981). For example, we may find it much more difficult to extricate ourselves from carrying out an order if we are partway through the process. This works on the principle that a small order is made first then followed by a moderate and subsequently a larger order. People are inclined to carry out the larger order once they have completed the smaller one. Milgram may have been criticised for the controversial and unethical nature of his experiments; however, he demonstrated clearly the extent to which people would go in order to obey authority. Moreover, it would be erroneous to believe that authority is the only source of social influence. Concepts such as conformity and compliance show a different dimension of social influence without orders from authority.

Conformity and compliance

To conform means to change one's behaviour in keeping with the behaviour of other group members. Conformity is based on group pressure, which can be real or imagined. Compliance on the other hand is changing our behaviour as a result of a direct request from someone who has no authority over us. For example, someone asks us to let them pass, we oblige and in doing so we would have complied with his or her request.

Why do we conform and comply?

There are at least five possible explanations as to why individuals would conform to the wishes of others, and these can be explained through the notions of public conformity, private acceptance, motivation to be liked, reward and punishment, and motivation to be correct. Public conformity suggests that in doing as others do individuals don't really change their minds or beliefs. Instead, they go along with the behaviour of others simply because it would seem socially desirable at the time. Private acceptance on the other hand is more about lack of conviction in people's own judgement. Therefore they come to perceive their own answers as inaccurate. Motivation to be liked can be linked with Maslow's (1970) self-esteem needs (see Chapter 1). Maslow (1970) describes esteem needs as one of the basic of human needs that contributes to the 'feeling of self-confidence, worth, strength, capacity, and adequacy, of being useful and necessary in the world' (p. 45). Reward and punishment as a way to seek conformity is based on Thorndike's (1911) concept of law of effect (see Chapter 5), the principle of which states that if a particular behaviour is rewarded it will most likely be repeated whereas a behaviour that is followed by discomfort will not. Discomfort in the context of this discussion is taken to mean punishment. It would seem that individuals' conformity is also driven by the need and motivation to be correct (see Insko et al., 1985). The definition of *correctness* rests with a group norm that tends to dictate what is right and what is wrong. An individual needs to be correct is so powerful that he or she has a tendency to agree even if the group norm is unmistakably wrong as indicated in Solomon Asch's (1952) classic study.

Asch (1958) was in effect trying to establish the 'social and personal conditions that induce individuals to resist or to yield to group pressures when the latter perceived to be *contrary to fact*' (p. 174). One of Asch's studies involved eight participants, seven of whom were confederates. For simplicity of explanation let us assume that participant number six was the true subject who was presented with two contradictory and conflicting sets of information. For example, he was faced with evidence of his own perception (senses) and that of a group of seven members. Participant number six thought that he was taking part in a study that involved visual perception. All participants were informed that they would be shown four lines (Figure 3.1), a standard line (A) and three other lines of varying lengths (X, Y, Z). Their task was to say out aloud, each in turn, which of the three lines (X, Y, and Z) was the same length as the standard line (A).

The experiment was structured so that the confederates were primed to give the same wrong answer at a predetermined trial (for example, trial number 3). Basically, the true subject (participant six) found himself in a situation whereby seven people highlighted standard line A as being equal in length to line Z when he clearly saw line Y as being the closest. Here we have a situation where seven people were unanimous in contradicting the evidence of one person. It begs the question, *if we were in the place of that one man how would we have reacted to this situation?* According to Asch's (1952) findings, a good number of us would most probably do what participant number six did and that is going against his own judgement and conviction by agreeing with others. In fact, out of 12 trials the subject went along with the majority in at least four trials. Moreover, about three-quarter of the subjects made at least one conforming response in the 12 trials.

Asch (1958) offers an illustration of one subject who despite group pressure remained independent and non-yielding. However, when the true nature of the experiment was disclosed to the subject, he commented that he felt happy and

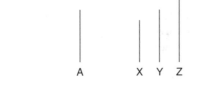

Figure 3.1   An example of Asch's (1952) set of line lengths.

relieved but added that he could not deny that at times he felt 'to heck with it, I'll go along with the rest' (Asch, 1958, p. 178). One could take this to imply that the power of social influence can be such that it can lead even the most confident person to the verge of succumbing to group pressure. In relation to the description of one subject who went with the majority in 11 out of 12 trials, Asch (1958) states, 'he appeared nervous and somewhat confused, but he did not attempt to evade discussion; on the contrary, he was helpful and tried to answer to the best of his ability' (Asch, 1958, p. 178). This particular subject; however, remarked that he would have probably responded differently had he offered his answer first. According to Asch (1958), 'this was his way of stating that he had adopted the majority estimates. The primary factor in his case was loss of confidence' (Asch, 1958, p. 178). Exercise 6 attempts to translate the notion of conformity to clinical practice.

EXERCISE 6

Reflect on your own clinical area, think of some examples where conformity was displayed.

Asch's experiments clearly show how people behaved in a norm that had already been established. From what has been presented so far it would seem that most of us would adopt the norm behaviour even if this is erroneous. Would we conform as easily when the norm has not been previously established? According to Sherif (1937) when a group of people are together they tend to establish a group norm that is maintained by an individual even in the absence of the group. Sherif used the autokinetic effect to support his point. Autokinetic effect is said to take place when a person perceives a fixed point of light shone onto a wall in a darkened room to move. Obviously, the movement of the light is not real and as a result the distance that the light seems to move varies from person to person. However, when placed in a group, Sherif found that members converged on group norms that were very strong and persistent. Even when members were separated from the group they reported the same shift as the group. The implication is that individuals have a strong tendency to conform to group norm regardless of their personal belief.

A theoretical understanding of the power of authority may lead to our awareness of when we are acting according to our own set of beliefs and values and when we are embracing authority's etiquette of submission by simply following orders. It could be said that carrying out one's duty without questioning its purpose and validity can only lead to, what Milgram (1974) calls, the perils of obedience. However, within a culture steeped in the medical model of care, how realistic is it for other health care professionals to question the credibility of medical prescription? As previously stated, the relationship between patients and health care professionals is asymmetrically positioned in favour of health care professionals. However, the vision of the National Health Service is to embrace the concept of partnership and collaboration in care where the aim is to read-dress this imbalance of power thus allowing patients to become true partners. In fact, the word 'empowerment' is now a great buzz word (Peterson, 2001) and fashionable in health care organisation (Gomm, 1993) that it almost feels surreal and we may risk looking like *fools rushing in*. We should really reflect what empowerment in a health care context truly means before embarking on a grandiose plan of *power to patient*.

Health care system: An empowering or disempowering process

What does it mean to empower? As with power, perhaps we should start with exploring the word empowerment itself (see Exercise 7).

EXERCISE 7

Make a list of all the words that come to mind when you hear the word 'empowerment'.

Exploring your list, try and deduce a common sentiment (or sentiments) that these words convey to you.

From what you have deduced thus far, define what you understand by the term empowerment.

According to Rappaport (1987), empowerment is a process whereby people gain mastery over their affairs. Gaining mastery of the situation indicates an intrapersonal dimension of empowerment (see Chapter 7). For example, individuals cognitively appraise their situation in terms of their capacity to influence it. Take another look at your list from Exercise 6 (see also Appendix 2), you may have noticed that almost every word carries a positive connotation. This would probably explain health professionals' eagerness to embrace the empowerment concept within health care. By definition therefore empowerment conveys a psychological sense of being in control, and the idea of empowering others suggests a process that enables individuals to have more control or influence over their own life. Moreover, in a health care context this would imply being able to influence to a large extent the type of care one receives. In fact, Sir Nigel Crisp, the then Chief Executive of the NHS states, 'our aim is that every patient should "feel tall" when they are cared for by the NHS' (DoH, 2005a, p. iii). The criteria for feeling tall seem to rest with an improved patients' emotional experience achieved through the following.

- Getting good treatment in a comfortable, caring, and safe environment, delivered in a calm and reassuring way.

- Having information to make choices, to feel confident, and to feel in control.

- Being talked to and listened to as an equal.

- Being treated with honesty, respect, and dignity (DoH, 2005a, pp. 64–65).

Thus far the Department of Health's (2005b) aim of making patient feel tall, especially the elderly, would appear to be a distant dream as evidence suggests that the standard of health care services is far from acceptable. For example, a joint report from the three public sector watchdogs, the Audit Commission, Healthcare Commission, and Commission for Social Care Inspection, reveals that discrimination exists in mental health services (Commission for Healthcare Audit and Inspection, 2006). Moreover, ageism 'ranges from patronising and thoughtless treatment from staff, to the failure of some mainstream public services such as transport, to take the needs and aspirations of older people seriously. Many older people find it difficult to challenge ageist attitudes and their reluctance to complain can often mean that nothing changes' (Commission for Healthcare Audit and Inspection, 2006, p. 7).

A further dimension inherent within the notion of empowerment is the process of educating and demystifying issues by raising what Jacob (1996) calls the population's collective consciousness. Implicit within raising patients' collective consciousness is the concept of 'informed choices'. Informed choice suggests interactional empowerment that emphasises interpersonal communication that leads to mastery over one's situation. The underlying principle in a health care context is that the clearer we are about a specific form of treatment, the easier it is for us to accept or refuse it. In practice, however, this is much more complex, and informed choices depend very much on health professionals' views of the phenomenon. For example, Peterson (2001) found that despite being compassionate and competent, many health care professionals showed disregard to patients' experiential knowledge, thus reinforcing their professional dominance. There are clear instances where patients were coerced into accepting the views of practitioners. Peterson (2001) states that on the face of it, empowerment appears to offer the promise of active participation of people with chronic illness in disease management. However, in reality evidence seems to point towards health professionals' incongruent behaviour manifested through the traditional biomedical model that contradicts the very essence of empowerment.

It could be said that in order to empower others one needs to be empowered. From Figure 3.2, it is clear that ultimate power in health service delivery lies with the Secretary of State through both policy making and control of funds. The Department of Health is helped by two bodies: the National Institute for Health and Clinical Excellence (responsible for setting standards for delivery of health services) and the Healthcare Commission (responsible for enforcing these standards). Power is devolved through to the Strategic Health Authorities responsible for managing, monitoring, and improving services at local level. Two of the principal players are NHS administrators and physicians. It could be argued that previous NHS administrators existed as agents for physicians in a passive alliance, facilitating their practice by solving problems, smoothing conflicts, and generally maintaining the organisation (Harrison, 1988). Contemporary health

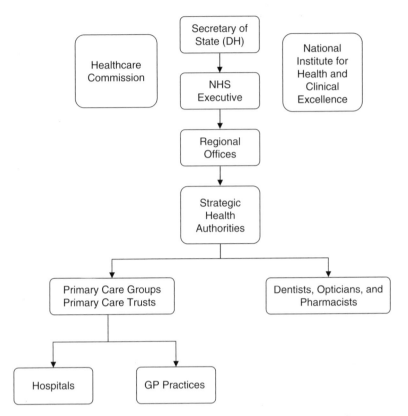

Figure 3.2 The hierarchical structure of the British National Health Service.

service organisation sees managers as having much greater formal power to control health care professionals as well as improving the quality of services provided. Learmonth (1999) suggests that improved management has led to the transformation of the health service for the good of all. Despite this, managers are perceived as controlling, oppressing, and mistrusting of their staff. At the point of health service delivery; therefore, clinicians ought to have power in order to empower patients. In the majority of cases this is not found to be the case. In mental health nursing, for example, Rungapadiachy (2006) found that some nurses felt unsupported, principally by managers above ward level and consultant psychiatrists. One participant in fact said, 'the team is very supportive to ward manager level. Beyond that it tends to be a bit of a blame culture' (Rungapadiachy, 2006, p. 537). However, looking at the hierarchy in context of the larger organisation (Figure 3.2) this *blame culture* may be the sign of a ripple effect from the Government. For example, Bradshaw (2002) argues that the system of health service delivery creaks under the weight of Government reform, and when things go wrong there is one particular target group to blame and that is the NHS managers. Similarly, when things go wrong at the point of health service delivery the target group for blame appears to be those on the shop floor, and if all else fails blame the doctors.

It could be argued that health service delivery is based on the notion of team-work (Herrman, Trauer, & Warnock, 2002). The implication is that members from each health care discipline would work in collaboration and support of each other in order to offer what is best for the patients. For example, Beni-erakis (1995) argues that a team can produce more and better work than its individual members working in isolation. According to Freeman, Miller, and Ross (2000), multi-professional teamwork has become the preferred model of practice promoted for many areas of health care by policy makers, professional bodies, and trust management (Calman & Hine, 1995; DoH, 1955, 1997, 1998; SCOPME, 1997). However, Rungapadiachy (2006) found a general feeling of lack of support experienced by most of his participants (mental health nurses), and this was identified as a source of frustration and stress, especially when faced with physicians who were not prepared to listen to them. Moreover, confront-ation between mental health nurses and doctors was non-existent because the former perceived this to be futile (interactional disempowerment). There was an implicit understanding on the part of mental health nurses who they were in a state of learned helplessness (see Chapter 2). Hence, it would seem that clinicians at lower levels are still caught into the subservient role where all they can do is carry out orders. This raises the question of *how feasible is it for clinicians on the shop floor to act as a patient's agent of empowerment, that is, as an advocate?* Clinicians who occupy a subservient role may not always be the best person to advocate for the patients principally because they have to conform to the judge-ment of their superiors. Moreover, as Willard (1996) says, the rigorous demands of advocacy make it unlikely that such a practitioner will be in a position to fulfil satisfactorily this obligation because advocacy is much more than speaking to other colleagues and other disciplines on a patient's behalf. Willard (1996) goes on to say that, from a legal perspective, advocacy would suggest that the person representing the patient has sufficient knowledge, power, and authority to make a difference to what may happen to the latter. As far as subservient practitioners are concerned this may prove difficult as they may have the knowledge but not the power and the authority to influence the judgement of their superiors.

The myth of patient power

'When will a sick note from a non-orthodox medicine practitioner become acceptable for sick pay' (Callinas-Correia, 2001)[4] The answer would perhaps explain why the belief that patient power is a myth. Callinas-Correia (2001) argues that the power of medicine arises out of the ownership of the model of reality where the patient accepts the primacy of the medical view of the world thus implying that doctors have the upper hand. Moreover, 'to accept the medical version of the patient's life implies the power of medicine upon the patient, exercised by the doctor. To consult an expert is to accept this state of affairs' (Callinas-Correia, 2001). One could not argue with this unless of course when the expert has a vested interest. However, Callinas-Correia acknowledges caution against accepting medical advice. 'The doctor may give less than optimal advice, as doctors are no longer independent advisers, but advisers employed to promote the excellence of their employer – the NHS' (Callinas-Correia, 2001). It is possible that patients are nothing but pawns in the interplay between government and doctors. For example, the government's idea of shifting the balance of power from doctors in favour of patients makes little sense, as Chinthapalli (2001) states that a doctor has more knowledge as well as having an obligation to the taxpayer. Taking doctors' power away would result in the destruction of medicine. Based on this discussion and by virtue of definition, it could be argued that patients will always be the least powerful group of people regardless of health care professionals' aim to embrace the concept of patient-centred care. The hierarchical system that we live in still places recipients of health services at the lowest rung of the ladder, principally because it is they who seek health services. The general rule in the patient-health care organisation is that those who 'seek' are always weaker than those who 'provide'. In a health care context it would seem that patient power might be a myth as patients may never be in a position to get what they want. A case in point is the disempowering circumstance in the provision of dental care in Britain where people are, to some extent, forced to seek private care because dentists are opting out of the NHS system. In this instance individuals have very little choice as they can either follow the dentists into private care or go without dental treatment. Going without dental treatment is not an option because of the health risk and the discomfort that this brings. Lack of choices would appear to be a primary cause for creating a power imbalance in the first instance, and yet the British Government emphasises that the 'NHS has now the capacity and capability to move on from being an organisation which simply delivers services to people to being one which is totally patient-led – responding to their needs and wishes' (DoH, 2005a, p. 5). Moreover, every aspect of the new system is designed to be patient led, where people have a far greater range of choices and information and help to make choices (see Exercise 8).

EXERCISE 8

Reflect on your clinical experience and identify instances where patients have choices in what they are involved in.

It may be difficult to come up with a comprehensive list because the instances where patients have choices could be few and far between. There are instances, however, where health service users have expressed their choice of treatment only to be told they can't have it because it costs too much. In this case, it would be wrong to believe that doctors are the only culprits in enforcing their power over patients, thus depriving them of their choice of treatment. For example, some Primary Care Trusts (PCT) in England have refused to treat some women who suffer from breast cancer with Herceptin. A case in point was that of Elaine Barber, a mother of four who was initially refused the drug despite her doctor's recommendation that she should be treated with it. Here, freedom of choice is constrained by economic barriers, thus making patient power as elusive and perhaps as mythical a concept as ever. On a positive note, however, this particular PCT reversed its decision and Elaine Barber who had threatened to take the PCT to court over its decision to deny her the drug was granted the treatment before the case went to court. It could be argued that in this instance, Elaine Barber was successful in exercising power through her right. However, this was at the cost of enduring personal stress as Ms. Barber felt that she was put through all this just so the health authority can balance the books. Moreover, there are many women who were not as lucky as Ms. Barber.

Both the Government and health care professionals' paternalistic attitude can serve as another barrier to patients exercising their choices. For example, in Britain patients can't exercise their right to die with dignity, instead they have to seek this service abroad as was the case with Dr. Anne Turner who suffered from supranuclear palsy, a progressive and incurable degenerative disease. Dr. Turner went to the Dignitas clinic in Zurich where doctors gave her drugs with which to end her life (BBC News, 2006). Paternalistic attitude to care can also be perceived to extend to caring for people with mental health problems in the shape of the Mental Health Act (1983), where doctors and nurses have the right under various sections of the act to detain people who are deemed mentally unwell. Moreover, there are specific sections that give practitioners the right to enforce treatment against patients' wishes. Obviously, some would see this as *for the good of the patients,* and for all intent and purposes the underlying principles of the Mental Health Act (1983) aim to protect patients as well as the public. However, for those who are on the receiving end of the Act, it is unlikely that they will see this as a liberating experience, perhaps more so as a draconian measure of social control. The Mental Health Act (1983) was due to be replaced, but after more than seven years of consultation, the Health Minister announced that attempts to radically overhaul mental health law were abandoned only to be replaced by proposals for a Bill to amend the existing Act. Interestingly, this new Bill introduces the notion of supervised treatment in the community to ensure patients' adherence to treatment long after they have been discharged from hospital. This begs the question *what does patient power mean to someone who is prescribed this supervised treatment?* The most obvious answer could be that patient power is a contradiction in term. Evidence suggests that the Mental Health Act (1983) has been used as a draconian tool for social control as was illustrated in the case of woman referred to as 'S', who was 36 weeks pregnant, detained under Section 2 of the Act in order for a Caesarean section to be performed for the birth of her baby. Medical argument was that 'S' was diagnosed with severe preeclampsia[5] that posed a threat to both her health and that of her unborn baby (St. George's Healthcare NHS Trust v S, 1998). However, 'S' was said to be fully aware of the potential risks but still rejected medical advice on the principle that she wanted a natural birth. 'S' was admitted to a psychiatric hospital against her will where she was transferred (still against her will) to a second hospital. Her GP had diagnosed her as suffering from depression that was confirmed by doctors at the hospital. There was insufficient evidence to question her competence. Moreover, the hospital did not consult

S's lawyer but instead applied ex parte[6] to the High Court for a declaration that would dispense with S's consent to treatment. This was granted, and a Caesarean section was performed successfully. S was then discharged to the first hospital, where she discharged herself as soon as the detention order had expired. What was ironic, however, was the fact that at no point during her confinement was S offered treatment for her so-called depression.

S applied for a judicial review of her admission, transfer, detention, and treatment, as well as appealing against the declaration. Below are some of the grounds as to why the appeal was successfully held.

- As an adult of sound mind a pregnant woman was entitled to refuse medical treatment even if her life and that of her unborn child depended on it. Moreover, forcible invasive surgery (Caesarean section as was the case) could not be justified based on the needs of a foetus.

- Mental Health Act (1983) should not have been used to detain S against her will simply because her thinking was irrational or bizarre. The court found no evidence to suggest that S was detained either for assessment or treatment of a mental health problem but instead the Act was used to treat her physical condition. Moreover, as the law stands, a person detained under the Mental Health Act (1983) could not be forced to undergo medical procedures where these are unrelated to her mental health state, unless she did not have the ability to give her consent.

On the face of S's case it would seem that patient power won the day because her appeal was upheld. On close analysis, however, this is far from the truth because it still means that she was deprived of her wish for a natural delivery of her baby. The principal issue here is disempowerment through violation of her basic human rights.

Empowering patients through effective engagement

The notion of engagement is discussed fully in Chapter 9, however, for the benefit of this chapter, engagement is taken to mean involving patients in their own care. Although it has been argued that patient power is nothing but an oxymoron it could be said that as educationalist and health care practitioner one has both a moral obligation and a professional responsibility to ensure that the transition from *patienthood* to *personhood* offers opportunities and avenues for patients to have as much control as possible (whenever appropriate) in the way they are cared for. To this end and with a particular model of care in mind (see Chapter 9) the focus is on how to empower patients. A proposed formula for an empowered practitioner is practitioner's self-knowledge and knowledge of theory of empowerment and disempowerment. The emphasis is very much on being aware of both the impact of the phenomena of empowerment and disempowerment on self. However, self-knowledge needs to be supplemented by theoretical knowledge of relevant concepts, for example, the dynamic of patient–practitioner interaction. It could be argued that only then will practitioners be able to empower patients. Exercise 9 emphasises the theme of self-awareness in relation to the concept of disempowerment.

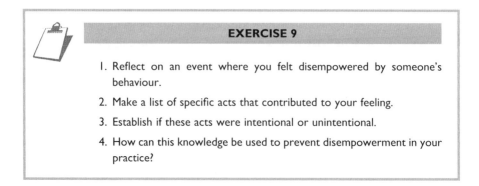

EXERCISE 9

1. Reflect on an event where you felt disempowered by someone's behaviour.

2. Make a list of specific acts that contributed to your feeling.

3. Establish if these acts were intentional or unintentional.

4. How can this knowledge be used to prevent disempowerment in your practice?

A deliberate action on the part of a practitioner that disempowers a client is seen as a perverted intervention. However, where the disempowering action is unintentional, the practitioner is perceived as degenerate (Heron, 2001). One possible explanation for degenerate practitioners is their lack of self-awareness. Reflecting on Exercise 9, it could be argued that if practitioners are able to capture and make sense of their feelings, thoughts, and actions during an encounter that is perceived as disempowering then they would be in a much better position to empathise with others who are enduring similar experience. Hence, communication may be much more effective. In Exercise 10, self-awareness relates to the notion of empowerment.

EXERCISE 10

Describe an encounter with another person where you felt empowered.
Describe a second encounter where you empowered another person.
Critically explore both these events and highlight all the empowering behaviour.
Reflect on how it feels to be empowered as well as how it feels to empower others.

We may feel an internal locus of control[7] when we are empowered in a given situation. Similarly, we may feel a sense of achievement when we have helped someone to regain his or her independence and autonomy. It could be argued that empowering starts with getting to know the other person, and as explained in Chapter 1, this process is facilitated by self-awareness.

How can patients be empowered? The answer rests with effective communication and in particular listening to them because only then will we be able to understand their individual needs. Therefore, from a health care practitioner's perspective, empowering behaviour needs to focus on our interpersonal styles of communication. According to Curtis and Diamond (1997), decreasing negative perception and increasing self-esteem may facilitate empowering behaviour. This implies that we should have as one of our assumptions that people are inherently good and that the basic needs, the basic human emotions, and the basic human capacities as they appear are neutral, premoral, or positively good (Maslow, 1999). Philosophies of care should always be underpinned by the need to recognise the patient as a human being first and foremost. This would serve to lead practitioners to acknowledge what Curtis and Diamond (1997) call 'the very real expertise of a person with a disability' and that 'can influence their power from position and expertise, as well as increase their personal power within the group' (p. 101). The need to acknowledge patients as expert appears to be fundamental to the notion of empowerment because they are the people with the real experience of illness and disability. To quote Curtis and Diamond (1997), 'as a psychiatrist, part of my expertise is knowing about psychotropic medications. As a medication user, knowing how a medication makes me feel is part of my expertise' (p. 102). Hence, the empowerment process rests with getting to know the patients first and foremost.

Summary

Implicit within the definition of power is the notion of influence, and having power means being able to control what one does. Power can be seen as a dispositional concept by virtue of the position one occupies. For example, the president of United States of America is regarded by some as the most powerful person in the world probably because he can carry out his own will despite resistance. Two dimensions of power are identified as 'power to', for example, having the ability to perform an act and 'power over' suggests possessing the ability to influence another person's behaviour. Some of the characteristics of power include intentionality, effectiveness, potentiality, and asymmetry. The power holder always has an asymmetrical relationship with the power object. Reflecting on the hierarchy in the NHS, it seems clear that consumers of health services are situated at the lowest rung of the ladder and as such could be perceived as least powerful. The implication is that they hold a deferential attitude towards health care professionals. The legitimacy of health care professionals' role together with the nature of the social situation contributes to the phenomenon of obedience. The aim of the NHS is to empower its consumers through freedom of treatment choice and autonomy. There is clear evidence to suggest that consumers are being denied of their choice of treatment for financial reasons. However, as health care professionals, we have a responsibility to try and ensure, through effective engagement, people's transition from patient to person and offers them opportunities and avenues to have as much control as possible in the care they receive. Effective engagement can be achieved through knowledge of theory and knowledge of self. Health care professionals need to be mindful of the fact that they may be experts in prescribing and administering treatment but it is the person enduring the problem who remains the expert in knowing how it feels to be empowered or disempowered depending on their lived experience.

References

Asch, S. E. (1952). *Social Psychology*. New York: Prentice Hall, Inc.

Asch, S. E. (1958). Effects of group pressure upon the modification and distortion of judgments. In E. Maccoby, T. M. Newcomb, and E. L. Hartley (eds.), *Readings in Social Psychology* (3rd edition, pp. 174–183). New York: Holt, Rinehart, and Wilson.

BBC 6 O'Clock News (2006). *Clinic Assists Doctor's Suicide*, Tuesday, 24 January.

Benierakis, C. E. (1995). The function of the multidisciplinary team in child psychiatry – clinical and educational aspects. *Canadian Journal of Psychiatry*, 40, 348–353.

Bierstedt, R. (1974). *Power and Progress: Essays on Sociological Theory*. New York, McGraw-Hill.

Blau, P. M. (1964). *Exchange and Power in Social Life*. New York and London: Wiley.

Blau, P. M. (1967). The hierarchy of authority in organizations. *American Journal of Sociology*, 73, 453–467.

Bradshaw, L. (2002). Managers, blame culture and highly ambitious policies in the British National Health Service (NHS). *Journal of Nursing Management*, 10, 1–4.

Callinas-Correia, J. (2001). What power for whom? *British Medical Journal*, 323(7310), 414. Available at http://www.bmj.com/cgi/eletters/323/7310/414.

Calman, K. and Hine, D. (1995). *A Policy Framework for Commissioning Cancer Services: A Report by the Expert Advisory Group on Cancer to the Chief Medical Officers of England and Wales*. London: Department of Heath.

Canter, R. (2001). Patients and medical power. *British Medical Journal*, 323, 414.

Chinthapalli, R. (2001). Power and duty. *British Medical Journal*, 323(7310), 414. Available at http://www.bmj.com/cgi/eletters/323/7310/414.

Commission for Healthcare Audit and Inspection (2006). *Living Well in Later Life: A Review of Progress Against the National Service Framework for Older People*. London: Commission for Healthcare Audit and Inspection.

Curtis, L. C. and Diamond, R. (1997). Power and coercion in mental health practice. In B. Blackwell (ed.), *Treatment Compliance and the Therapeutic Alliance* (pp. 97–122). The Netherlands: Harwood Academic Publishers.

Department of Health (1955). *A Policy Framework for Commissioning Cancer Services: A Report by the Expert Advisory Group on Cancer to the Chief Medical Officers of England and Wales*. London: Department of Health.

Department of Health (DoH) (1997). *The New NHS: Modern and Dependable*. London: HMSO.

Department of Health (1998). *A First Class Service: Quality in the NHS*. London: HMSO.

Department of Health (2001). *Involving Patients and the Public in Healthcare: A Discussion Document*. London: Department of Health.

Department of Health (2005a). *Creating a Patient-Led NHS: Delivering the NHS Improvement Plan*. London, Department of Health.

Department of Health (2005b). *'Now I Feel Tall' What a Patient-Led NHS Feels LIKE*. London: Department of health.

Dowding, K. (1996). *Power*. Buckingham: Open University Press.

Freeman, M., Miller, C., and Ross, N. (2000). The impact of individual philosophies of teamwork on multi-professional practice and the implications for education. *Journal of Interprofessional Care*, 14(3), 237–247.

French, J. R. P. and Raven, B. H. (1959). The bases of social power. In D. Cartwright (ed.), *Studies in Social Power* (pp. 150–167). Ann Arbor: Institute for Social Research.

Gilbert, S. J. (1981). Another look at Milgram obedience studies. The role of the graduated series of shocks. *Personality and Social Psychology Bulletin*, 7, 690–695.

Goffman, E. (1961). *Asylums: Essays on the Social Situation of Mental Patients and Other Inmates.* Garden City, NY: Penguin Books.

Gomm, R. (1993). Issues of power in health and welfare. In J. Walmsley, J. Reynold, P. Shakespear, and R. Woolfe (eds.), *Health Welfare and Practice* (pp. 131–138). London: Sage Publication.

Harrison, S. (1988). *Managing the NHS: Shifting the Frontier?* London: Chapman & Hall.

Heron, J. (2001). *Helping the Client: A Creative Practical Guide.* London: Sage.

Herrman, H., Trauer, T., and Warnock, J. (2002). The roles and relationships of psychiatrists and other service providers in mental health services. *Australian and New Zealand Journal of Psychiatry*, 2002: 36: 75–80.

Hunter, M. (2001). News: Alder Hey report condemns doctors, management, and coroner. *British Medical Journal*, 322, 255.

Insko, C. A., Smith, R. H., Alicke, M. D., Wade, J., and Taylor, S. (1985). Conformity and group size. *Personality and Social Psychology Bulletin*, 11, 41–50.

Jacob, F. (1996). Empowerment: a critique. *British Journal of community Health Nursing*, 1(8), 449–453.

Learmonth, M. (1999). The National Health Service manager, engineer and father? A deconstruction. *Journal of Management Studies*, 36(7), 999–1012.

Maslow, A. H. (1970). *Motivation and Personality.* New York, Evanston, and London: Harper and Row Publishers.

Maslow, A. H. (1999). *Toward a Psychology of Being* (3rd edition). New York: John Wiley and Sons, Inc.

Mental Health Act (1983). Chapter 20. London: H.M.S.O.

Milgram, S. (1963). Behavioural study of obedience. *Journal of Abnormal and Social Psychology*, 67, 371–378.

Milgram, S. (1965). Liberating effects of group pressure. *Journal of personality and Social Psychology*, 1, 127–134.

Milgram, S. (1974). *Obedience to Authority: An Experimental View.* London: Tavistock Publications Ltd.

Parsons, T. (1951). *The Social System.* Glencoe: The Free Press.

Parsons, T. (1975). The sick role and the role of the physician reconsidered. *Millbank Memorial Fund Quarterly*, 53, 257–278.

Peterson, B. (2001). Myth of empowerment in chronic illness. *Journal of Advanced Nursing*, 34(5), 574–581.

Rappaport, J. (1987). Terms of empowerment/exemplars of prevention: toward a theory for community psychology. *American Journal of Community Psychology*, 15(2), 121–148.

Rogers, C. R. (1946). Significant aspects of client-centered therapy. *American Psychologist*, 1, 415–422.

Rungapadiachy, D. M. (2006). How newly qualified mental health nurses perceive their role. *Journal of Psychiatric and Mental Health Nursing*, 13, 533–542.

SCOPME (1997). Multiprofessional working and learning: sharing the educational challenge. *The Standing Committee on Postgraduate Medical and Dental Consultation Paper*, London.

Sherif, M. (1937). An experimental approach to the study of attitudes. *Sociometry*, 1, 90–98.

St. George's Healthcare NHS Trust v S; R v Collins and other ex parte S (1998) *FLR* 728.

Thorndike, E. L. (1911). *Animal Intelligence: Experimental Studies.* New York, Macmillan.

Turner, J. C. (2005). Explaining the nature of power: a three-process theory. *European Journal of Social Psychology* 35, 1–22.

Weber, M. (1947). *The Theory of Social and Economic Organization.* New York: Oxford University Press.

Willard, C. (1996). The nurse's role as patient advocate: obligation or imposition? *Journal of Advanced Nursing*, 24, 60–66.

Wrong, D. (1979). Power. *Its Forms, Bases and Uses.* Oxford: Basil Blackwell.

Emotion of Loss and Self-Awareness

Dev M. Rungapadiachy

After reading this chapter you should be able to

.

- Discuss the concept of loss and grief.

- Demonstrate through self-awareness your understanding of the emotional response to loss in self and others.

- Discuss the process of managing loss and grief in self and others.

Introduction

One could argue that the meaning of loss as perceived by individuals is fundamental to their coping strategies and is thus crucial to the healing process. From a social constructionist point of view, the grieving process is both a voyage of healing as well as a rebuilding of meaning and representations of self (Hsu et al., 2004). It could be said that the impact of loss on an individual depends on various factors, for example, the value or significance of the loss object and the depth of emotional attachment associated with that object. Loss and grief therefore need to be viewed as an individual experience. The implication is that understanding the multifaceted concepts of loss and grief with the various coping strategies becomes central to health service delivery. This chapter explores the concepts of loss and grief in relation to understanding and managing one's own loss as well as helping others to deal with their losses. The starting point, however, is with definitions of terms.

Definition of terms

For simplicity of discussion, loss can be described as an emotion that is aroused as a result of separation from an object of attachment.[1] Grief is a natural response to the loss object and is displayed emotionally, physically, and socially. Grief reaction can also be anticipatory, for example when a loss is expected an individual may start grieving before the loss has actually occurred. Once the loss has taken place, an individual will still display grieving behaviour. Anticipatory grief is seen as a normal phenomenon. Bereavement is the experience of grieving that Parkes (1982) considers to be individually defined, thus individuals will display their grief in various ways. Mourning is the period during which grief response is displayed. However, Richards (1984) states that mourning can mean both the affect of grief and its outward manifestation. Moreover, Engel (1961) believes mourning is a process that takes time until restoration of function occurs.

The concept of loss

Loss, as previously defined, is an emotion that is aroused as a result of separation from an object of attachment. However, the concept of loss is much more complicated than this definition suggests. One does not necessarily have to be attached to the object in order to experience a sense of loss. For example, the expectation of being promoted to a higher status or position but not actually getting promotion would also result in a sense of loss. Moreover, loss can be real or imagined. A *real loss* is actual and may have already occurred (for example, death) or is imminent (for example, redundancy). *Imagined loss* can be seen as a misinterpretation or false perception of being separated from one's object of attachment (for example, the imagined potential of having a life-threatening illness as sometimes the case with someone suffering from anxiety). In both instances, individuals experience a sense of loss. Numerous words or phrases are often used to convey the sentiment of loss as can be seen from Exercise 1.

EXERCISE I

This exercise has two parts.

1. Brainstorm the word loss.

2. Explore each of the words you have identified in greater detail and explain their relationship with loss.

Numerous words associated with loss can be found in Appendix 3. Note the word *missing*, and in an attempt to explain the relationship with loss *missing* can be taken to mean *I miss you*. The implication here is that *I miss you* because *you are not where you usually are*. There is a change in proximity, for example, the physical distancing between two people has increased and access to one another is not as it was and may be problematic. Although this may be temporary, one may still experience a sense of loss. According to Parkes (1972), loss is a way of life, for example, people encounter numerous changes during their lifetime and

> every change involves a loss and a gain. The old environment must be given up, the new accepted. People come and go; one job is lost, another begun; territory and possessions are acquired or sold; new skills are learnt, old abandoned; expectations are fulfilled or hopes dashed – in all those situations the individual is faced with the need to give up one mode of life and accept another.
>
> (Parkes, 1972, p. 11)

However, the need to accept life changes can be problematic depending on the nature or type of the loss, the depth of attachment one has with the loss object, and the type of person one is (see Chapter 2, 'Attributional Style' and 'Locus of Control').

The concept of attachment

For the purpose of this discussion, attachment is taken to mean a strong emotional bond or tie with an object. The word *object* is used deliberately in order to emphasise that attachment behaviour is not, as a general rule, reciprocal although it can be. As Cassidy (1999) says, 'this bond is not one between two people; it is instead a bond that one individual has to another individual . . .' (p. 12). For example, person A *feels attached to person B this does not mean that person B feels attached to person A.* Numerous theories have been proposed to explain the notion of attachment. However, the one predominantly used is that of Bowlby's (1982). Bowlby's theory emerged from ideas within several approaches including biological theories about preservation of species. Bowlby (1982) argues that both infants and mothers (or mother figures) develop a biological need to be together and this very need contributes to the survival of babies and infants because they are vulnerable and need protection for a considerable length of time after birth. According to Bowlby (1980), attachment behaviour is conceptualised as any activity that results in a person attaining or retaining proximity to some other differentiated and preferred person. Moreover as 'long as the attachment figure remains accessible and responsive the behaviour may consist of little more than checking by eye or ear on the whereabouts of the figure and exchanging occasional glances and greetings' (Bowlby, 1980, p. 39). Sucking, clinging, following, crying, and smiling are five important patterns of behaviour that 'between the ages of about nine and eighteen months they usually become incorporated into far more sophisticated goal-corrected systems. These systems are so organised and activated that a child tends to be maintained in proximity to his mother' (Bowlby, 1980, p. 180). It would appear also that children could have more than one attachment figure. Bowlby (1982) states that 'many children have more than one figure towards whom they direct attachment behaviour; these figures are not treated alike; the role of a child's principal attachment-figure can be filled by others than the natural mother' (p. 304). However, when children are distressed they prefer their mother (Cassidy, 1999). In this instance the mother is seen as the principal attachment figure. This strong tendency for the infants to prefer a principal attachment figure for comfort and security is called monotropy. The implication is that the depth of attachment in monotropy is far greater than in any other attachment figure.

Separation

Words or phrases such as *to be apart, to be physically disconnected*, and *to be by oneself* would all describe the notion of separation. By its very nature, separation causes a state of disequilibrium that requires an individual to adapt to the change. Bowlby's (1973) observation suggests that separation can have a detrimental effect on children for example, not only were they 'intensely possessive and jealous of their "own" nurse but they were also unusually prone to become hostile towards her or to reject her, or else to retreat into a state of emotional detachment' (p. 4). Bowlby concludes that the sequence of responses of children observed during their stays in institutional settings were as follows.

- Protest is the initial phase that can last for a few hours to a week or even more and starts the moment the attachment figures prepare to leave their children. This phase is demonstrated by loud crying or screaming and marked anger. Kobak (1999) remarks that any sight or sound might temporarily produce a respite as a result of the child's hyper vigilance in anticipating the return of the mother. Moreover, the child remains desperate to regain contact with the mother. However, any comforting interventions offered by others are met with resistance and hence have little success.

- Despair is characterised by a feeling of hopelessness about the mother's return, crying becomes intermittent, and the child may become withdrawn or disengaged from others. Bowlby (1973) states, 'provided the period of separation is not too prolonged, a child does not remain detached indefinitely. Sooner or later after being reunited with his mother his attachment to her emerges afresh' (p. 3). However, the child will tend to stay close to his or her mother and the fear of losing her again arouses acute anxiety.

- Detachment is the final phase in the sequence of behaviour as a result of a child's separation from his or her mother. During detachment, children were observed to turn their attentions to the environment as if ignoring their mothers. For example, referring to one child, Bowlby (1973) states, 'he seems to lose his interest in his mother and to become emotionally *detached* from her' (p. 26). Moreover, Kobak (1999) states that a child who reached the phase of detachment demonstrated a 'striking absence of joy at the mother's return; instead of enthusiastically greeting her, the detached child was likely to be apathetic' (p. 25).

Loss and grief

It would seem that most of the intense emotions are aroused during the formation, maintenance, disruption, and renewal of attachment relationship. For example, the 'formation of a bond is described as falling in love, maintaining a bond as loving someone, and losing a partner as grieving over someone' (Bowlby, 1980, p. 40). Moreover, the threat of loss leads to anxiety whereas the actual loss itself brings about sorrow. The principle question for us as health care practitioners (regardless of status) and educators is *when does grieving over a loss become problematic?* Before attempting to answer this question, it would be helpful to consider the nature and types of loss.

Types of loss

Loss can be clustered under various categories. Exercise 2 attempts to contextualise types of loss.

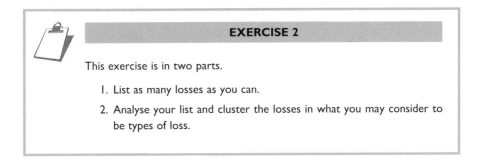

EXERCISE 2

This exercise is in two parts.

1. List as many losses as you can.

2. Analyse your list and cluster the losses in what you may consider to be types of loss.

A multidimensional approach

A multidimensional view of loss in the context of this chapter is confined to the five interrelated and overlapping themes of physical, emotional, intellectual, social, and spiritual. Physical dimension includes both an individual's anatomical organs and physiological functions.

Physical loss

Physical loss can be linked to material self,[2] and this can be divided into two categories: self and the environment. The loss of self can be explored from both an anatomical and a physiological perspective. Anatomical losses, some of which are highlighted in Figure 4.1, range from loss of hair to loss of limbs. Similarly, physiological losses range from loss of sight to loss of functions of the limbs (see Figure 4.2). Environmental loss includes any material possessions such as one's car, home, and wallet/purse.

Emotional loss

Emotional dimension of loss relates to an individual's feelings and words, such as mood and affect, that are used synonymously. However, mood can be seen

ANATOMICAL LOSS

Facial disfigurement

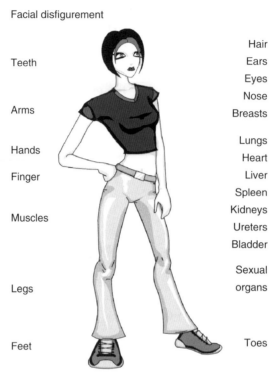

Teeth

Arms

Hands

Finger

Muscles

Legs

Feet

Hair

Ears

Eyes

Nose

Breasts

Lungs

Heart

Liver

Spleen

Kidneys

Ureters

Bladder

Sexual organs

Toes

Figure 4.1   Showing some anatomical losses.

PHYSIOLOGICAL LOSS

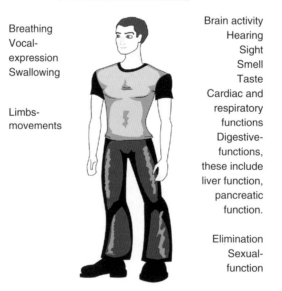

Breathing
Vocal-
expression
Swallowing

Limbs-
movements

Brain activity
Hearing
Sight
Smell
Taste
Cardiac and
respiratory
functions
Digestive-
functions,
these include
liver function,
pancreatic
function.

Elimination
Sexual-
function

Figure 4.2   Showing some physiological losses.

as a person's frame of mind, whilst affect refers to the outward display of emotions. It could also be said that both mood and affect are underpinned by feeling. Loss is the felt emotion as a result of separation from one's object of attachment and as such is most likely to be a reaction rather than a type of loss. However, it is not uncommon for people to complain of having lost their emotion as in feeling *numb, blunt, flat*, and *anhedonia*, described as the inability to experience pleasure from normally pleasurable events and characteristic of depression.

Intellectual loss

Intellectual dimension of loss focuses on cognitive functions that to a large extent are dictated by the physiological dimension. Exercise 3 asks for analytical thinking.

EXERCISE 3

Explore some of the anatomical and physiological losses highlighted in Figures 4.1 and 4.2 and establish the link between these and intellectual losses.

Intellectual loss can be assessed on people's ability to gain mastery over their situations. This would emphasise what they can or can't achieve cognitively, that is, sending and receiving information, memory, thinking, recollection of past events, and problem solving. In some cases, intellectual loss is underpinned by both anatomical and physiological loss. One such example is dementia, which is described as a chronic mental disorder characterised by deterioration of personality, confusion, disorientation,[3] and cognitive impairment such as loss of memory. Individuals with dementia, especially during the latter stage of development, often experience difficulty in communicating with others. Other types of intellectual loss include feeling *brain-drained* and loss of intellectual property.

Social loss

Social dimension relates to people's interaction with others, thus enabling them to function in society. Implicit within social dimension is the notion of inter-personal relationship and communication. Individuals exist in a dynamic state of interaction with the society they live in and as a result they learn to function within that particular society. You may have already identified from Exercise 1 some of the losses associated to the social dimension. Exercise 4 attempts to contextualise social loss.

EXERCISE 4

Reflect on Exercise I as well as the words associated with loss in Appendix 3 and tease out what you consider to be social losses and offer your rationale. For example, death of a loved one could be seen as a social loss because we will be deprived of their company. Hence, we miss not having them around.

Spiritual loss

Spiritual dimension embraces people's whole philosophy of life including their religion, culture, and political ideologies. Spiritual dimension often overlaps with both social and intellectual dimensions. For example, the very essence of one's philosophy is based on one's values and beliefs. Examples of loss of spirituality would include loss of faith, trust, beliefs, motivation, sense of self, and even the will to live.

Grief is a natural process

According to Engel (1961) 'grief is the characteristic response to the loss of a valued object, be it a loved person, a cherished possession, a job, status, home, country, an ideal, a part of the body, etc.' (p. 18). Provided it is uncomplicated, grief will run its natural course. Engel (1961), however, argues that, as with other diseases, grief fulfils all the criteria of a discrete syndrome, for example, it involves suffering, inhibits functions, is disabling, and leads to distress although these may be temporary. One can deduce from this that grieving is an illness and there may be some validity in Engel's sentiment provided, of course, one is prepared to consider the notion of illness from the perspective of the medical model. As Prior (1989) notes that historically the study of the grief reaction has been directed towards quantifying the individual's grief as a distinguishing *abnormal* reaction, as a consequence bereavement has become *medicalised*. It is worthwhile noting that grief does not always run its natural course and can instead become complicated. Complicated grief may require input from health care professionals, therefore in order to understand the notion of complicated grief reaction one would need to consider the so-called *normal grief reaction*. Grief as was previously stated is the emotional response to a loss and there are numerous theories that attempt to explain this phenomenon. A brief overview of the theories postulated by Bowlby (1980), Parkes (1972), and Kübler-Ross (1969) is offered here.

John Bowlby: Four phases of mourning

According to Bowlby (1980), people respond to the loss of a loved one by moving through a succession of phases. These phases are not straightforward, but individuals can move back and forth between any two of them and at any time. However, the process of mourning does follow an overall sequence, and these are highlighted in four phases.

Phase one: Numbing

Parallels could be drawn between physical numbing and emotional numbing. For example, individuals who have been stabbed often remarked that they felt no pain at the time of stabbing. According to Holmes (1993), a wounded soldier may feel no pain and carry on fighting until help is available. Similarly, the first reaction to the loss of a loved one may be that of emotional numbing where there is an 'emotional shutdown in which all feelings are suppressed, or reality denied, until the bereaved person is in a safe enough situation to let go a little' (Holmes, 1993, p. 90). Some individuals behave as though they are shocked, and it is this numbing phase that contributes to individuals' inability to accept the bad news. According to Bowlby (1980), for a time some individuals may continue with their life as if they are on automatic pilot. However, they will still feel tense, apprehensive, and may display an outburst of intense emotion in the forms of panic attacks or anger.

Phase two: Yearning, searching, and anger

This phase suggests that the reality of the loss is being gradually acknowledged. According to Bowlby (1980), 'this leads to pangs of intense pining and to spasms of distress and tearful sobbing' (p. 86). Some of the characteristics of the yearning phase are

- Restlessness

- Insomnia

- Preoccupation with the deceased often accompanied by feeling their actual presence

- Dreams of the deceased person as being still alive

- Misinterpretation of cues leading to the belief that the person has returned.

Bowlby (1980) emphasises these characteristics as normal, given that the majority of people would display these features. Moreover, anger is a common expression of the yearning phase, and in most cases, this is seen to be directed towards those believed to be responsible for the loss. Anger is also aroused as a result of frustrations from an individual's fruitless search for the lost object. According to Bowlby, mourning runs a healthy course with an intense urge to search and recover the loss. This intensity is greater in the early weeks and gradually diminishes over a period of time. Yearning and searching experience is believed to vary from individual to individual.

Phase three: Disorganisation and despair

Bowlby sees disorganisation and despair as a requisite for a favourable outcome of successful grieving.

> Only if he can tolerate the pining, the more or less conscious searching, the seemingly endless examination of how and why the loss occurred, and anger at anyone who might have been responsible, not sparing even the dead person, can he come gradually to recognize and accept that the loss is in truth permanent and that his life must be shaped anew.
>
> (Bowlby, 1980, p. 93)

Disorganisation is the phase during which old ways of behaving need to be relinquished before new ones can be assimilated, and this automatically leads to despair, depression, and apathy.

Phase four: Reorganisation

During the reorganisation phase, individuals begin to explore their new situation and contemplate ways of dealing with it. The implication is that individuals need to redefine themselves in the context of their new situation and only then will they be able to move on. Reorganisation involves taking on new roles, which means learning new skills, and according to Bowlby (1980), the more successful individuals are in achieving these new roles and skills, the more confident and independent they begin to feel.

Colin Murray-Parkes: Phases of grieving

> Losses are, of course, common in all our lives. And in so far as grief is the reaction to loss, grief must be common too. But the term grief is not normally used for the reaction to the loss of an old umbrella. It is more usually reserved for the loss of a person, and a loved person at that.
>
> (Parkes, 1996, p. 7)

The above quote suggests that Parkes (1996) is clear in terms of the very essence of grief, and true, one can't say that any loss will automatically lead to grief. Grief response is only manifested in relation to what could be seen as a significant loss. For example, the loss object needs to have meant something to an individual. Parkes (1971) posits that bereavement is a psychosocial transition in that loss poses a threat to one's inner assumptions about the world that leads to an emotional impact. This emotional impact is usually the consequence of disruption to one's life. When loss threatens an individual's security and stability, the grief felt is intense.

Parkes (1996) argues that grief is a process and not a state. Moreover, it is not 'a set of symptoms which starts after a loss and then gradually fades away' (Parkes, 1996, p. 7). Grief is instead a process consisting of at least five phases beginning with numbness through to pining, disorganisation, despair, and recovery. Parkes states that faced with a loss, an individual experiences numbness, which then gives way to pining and pining in turn gives way to disorganisation and despair. Recovery will only take place after the period of disorganisation is experienced.

Phase one: Numbness

The concept of numbness is as described in Bowlby's first phase of grieving. According to Parkes, numbness can occur soon after the news of the loss or even some minutes later and can last up to anything from a few hours to a few days. Numbness can be seen as an adaptive strategy in that it helps the individual to deal with the immediate need of the situation. Parkes (1972) states that 11 of his 22 London widows reported feeling numb or blunt. The numbness phase is manifested through outbursts of extreme distress and the bereaved person may even feel ill. Numbness is still experienced in cases where death came as a relief.

Phase two: Pining

The pining phase is similar to Bowlby's yearning and searching. Parkes (1996) refers to pining as the pangs of grief, which is an episode of severe anxiety and psychological pain. Pining is a subjective and emotional aspect of this desire to search for the loss and starts within a few hours or days of grieving reaching its maximum intensity within 5 to 14 days.

Phase three: Disorganisation

Pining gives way to disorganisation, and this phase is marked by depression when the individual may withdraw from contact with others. Here, feelings of despair and apathy are aroused. An individual will not be able to progress to recovery until disorganisation is overcome through the realisation that changes in attitude and behaviour are called for in order to make a new start.

Phase four: Recovery

The recovery phase is the period when realisation of the loss is clearly recognised and the need for change acknowledged. However, it would be wrong to think of the recovery phase as *getting over it* because people do not get over their loss, instead they get used to it. According to Parkes and Weiss (1983), recovery involves three distinct tasks and these are as follows.

- **The loss needs to be accepted intellectually**: Loss would seem to bring with it a sense of confusion and irrationality. For example, the bereaved person can't make sense of what is happening. According to Parkes and Weiss (1983), one of the functions of grieving is that it enables the person to make sense and understand their loss. Grieving allows some sort of explanation to be arrived at with regards to *why the death*.

- **The loss needs to be accepted emotionally**: One sign of emotional acceptance is when bereaved people are able to face events that remind them of their loss without feeling distraught. This task can be facilitated through repeated exposure to the reminders of the loss until such a time when there is a reduction in the intensity of painful emotion. Moreover, 'the pleasure of recollection begins to outweigh the pain' (Parkes & Weiss, 1983, p. 157).

- **The individual needs to change in congruence with the new reality**: Loss brings changes that require the bereaved person to adopt a change of attitude to the one previously held. For example, a married woman after losing her husband is no longer a married woman, but a widow instead. The woman needs to acknowledge this reality, and this, however, does not happen overnight. It is a long drawn out process but successful recovery demands for this change of attitude. Parkes and Weiss (1983) explain that 'the bereaved woman who insists that she is "Jack's wife and not Jack's widow," while expressing an admirable loyalty to her marriage, displays as well a commitment to an obsolete identity' (p. 159).

Elizabeth Kübler-Ross: Five stages of grieving

Kübler-Ross (1969) developed her model of grief based on interviews with over 200 terminally ill people and concluded that faced with their terminal illness, people adopt five coping strategies that begin with denial and isolation through to anger, bargaining, depression, and acceptance.

First stage: Denial and isolation

Denial, as discussed in Chapter 1, is a mental defence mechanism displayed as a reaction to some unpleasant event. Kübler-Ross found that most of her participants displayed initial denial when they were told of the nature of their illness. Verbal expressions of denial were in the form of 'no, not me, it cannot be true' (Kübler-Ross, 1969, p. 34). Moreover, people may want to seek for a second or third opinion in the hope that the initial diagnosis was inaccurate. Others may say *there is a mix up and this cannot be happening to me*. Kübler-Ross (1969) points out that denial is much more typical in patients who are 'informed prematurely or abruptly by someone who does not know the patient well or does it quickly "to get it over with" without taking the patient's readiness into consideration' (p. 35). Denial serves to cushion the painful and shocking news, thus allowing the person some sense of composure. It is seen as a temporary defence soon to be replaced by partial acceptance. Kübler-Ross states that much later the patient uses isolation more than denial. Exercise 5 helps to recognise some of the manifestations of denial.

EXERCISE 5

Denial, in the context of loss and grief, is an unconscious resistance or refusal to acknowledge the event has taken place. Identify some of the characteristics that may lead you to suspect that a grieving person is in denial?

A bereaved person's verbal communication can serve as a good indication of the state of denial. For example, if someone constantly refers to the deceased person in present tense then it is most likely that denial is at play. *Constantly* is emphasised because people could use present tense in error or as a force of habit in which case it would be wrong to assume a state of denial. Behaviourally, if a bereaved individual sets the dining table to include the deceased person (and again provided this is a persistent behaviour) then one can safely assume that he or she is in a state of denial.

Second stage: Anger

Denial gives way to a new set of reactions in the form of anger, rage, envy, and resentment. During this stage the bereaved person questions, *why me? Why couldn't it have been someone else?* Kübler-Ross states that anger is difficult to cope with especially for family and health care professionals because it is displaced in all directions and projected at random. The problem according to Kübler-Ross (1969) is that 'few people place themselves in the patient's position and wonder where this anger might come from' (p. 45). Exercise 6 helps to understand the rationale for a bereaved person's anger.

EXERCISE 6

Imagine you have been told that you have lost something or someone. Why might you display anger?

Kübler-Ross believes that the expression of anger on the part of the bereaved person may be one way of seeking recognition for still being alive. Some would argue that the source of anger might be frustration resulting from the sudden disruption to one's life. Moreover, reality may be too painful to have to adjust to. Anger therefore becomes one of the unconscious ways of behaving.

Third stage: Bargaining

If we have been unable to face the sad facts in the first period and have been angry at people and God in the second phase, maybe we can succeed in entering into some sort of an agreement which may postpone the inevitable happening: "If God has decided to take us from this earth and he did not respond to my angry pleas, he may be more favourable if I ask nicely"'.

(Kübler-Ross, 1969, p. 72)

The above quote captures the essence of bargaining. Here the bereaved person tries to make some sort of a pact with God in the hope that the latter will allow him or her special favour in the form of 'an extension of life, followed by the wish for a few days without pain or physical discomfort' (Kübler-Ross, 1969, p. 73).

Fourth stage: Depression

This stage would suggest that the bereaved person has come to realise that death is inevitable and much more a reality. Illness can no longer be denied, therefore depression is felt. Kübler-Ross considers two types of depression that terminally ill patients seem to endure. The first type, reactive depression, relates to the reaction to the loss while the second type, preparatory depression, is associated with patients' final preparation for their separation from the world. In reactive depression, the bereaved person responds not only to the loss of having been told of their condition but also to the added loss that their incapacitated state brings, for example loss of job and reduced financial income. On preparatory depression, Kübler-Ross states that it does not occur as a result of a past loss but does take into account impending losses.

Fifth stage: Acceptance

Acceptance is seen as the final stage of the grieving process and Kübler-Ross warns that this should not be mistaken for a happy stage. She adds that accept-ance is almost void of feelings. 'It is as if the pain had gone, the struggle is over' (Kübler-Ross, 1969, p. 100). The terminally ill person accepts that the end is near and loses interest in others and the environment with a wish to be left alone. Payne and Horn (1999) state that a terminally a ill person's withdrawal from others may be experienced as rejection and may be difficult to understand if family and friends are not ready to let go of the person.

All three writers, Bowlby, Parkes, and Kübler-Ross, have described people's responses to their own loss in terms of stages (see Table 4.1). Moreover, they expressed similar sentiments in terms of how people react when faced with a loss. However, these similarities seem more obvious between Bowlby and Parkes.

As far as stage theory goes, the implication is that people would start at one stage (numbness, denial, and isolation) and move their way through to the end point (reorganisation, recovery, and acceptance). However, it would be erroneous to assume this to be the case with one's reaction to a loss object. Given that loss is an individual experience, it can't be seen as a universal

Table 4.1 An overview of the stages of grieving from Bowlby (1980), Parkes (1972), and Kübler-Ross's (1969) perspectives

Phase/stage	Bowlby (1980)	Parkes (1972)	Kübler-Ross (1969)
One	Numbing	Numbness	Denial and isolation
Two	Yearning, searching, and anger	Pining	Anger
Three	Disorganisation and despair	Disorganisation	Bargaining
Four	Reorganisation	Recovery	Depression
Five			Acceptance

experience as stage theory would suggest. Kastenbaum (2000) makes a good point by saying that 'stage interpretation neglected the patients' total life situation, including, for example, relationship support and conflicts, family obligations, specific effects of their illness, and the management and communication milieu to which they were exposed (for example, an anxious and denying institutional climate)' (p. 223). Regardless of how one may feel about stage theories, what seems clear is that they do contribute to our knowledge of the concept of loss and its possible influence on behaviour. It is beyond the scope of this chapter to offer a critique of Bowlby, Parkes, and Kübler-Ross's works. Interestingly, however, despite the numerous criticisms, the espoused theory of Kübler-Ross (1969) is well used in health care courses (Down-Wamboldt & Tamlyn, 1997).

Mourning

Loss is said to disturb an individual's equilibrium, and mourning serves to readdress this imbalance. Rando (2000) sees mourning as both a conscious and unconscious process that serves to help the mourner to (a) detach from the object of attachment (b) adapt to the loss, and (c) exhibit coping behaviour in the absence of the loss object. The properties of these three clusters are highlighted as the 'six "R" processes of mourning' (Rando, 2000, p. 63): **R**ecognise the loss, **R**eact to the separation, **R**ecollect and reexperience the loss, **R**elinquish the old attachments, **R**eadjust to the new world without forgetting the old one, and lastly **R**einvest in another relationship. Most, if not all, of the six 'R' processes of mourning are addressed in the seminal work of Worden (1982) in the section that follows.

William Worden: The four tasks of mourning

According to Worden (1982), grief is a process and not a state. The implication is that bereaved individuals should work with their feeling and reaction to the loss instead of putting up resistances. Worden (1982) proposes four specific tasks that mourning serves and these are accept the reality of the loss, experience the pain of grief, adjust to an environment in which the deceased is missing, and withdraw emotional energy and reinvest it in another relationship.

Task one: Accepting the reality of the loss

It is clear from Bowlby (1980), Parkes (1972), and Kübler-Ross (1969) that when someone dies the bereaved person initially feels a sense of shock, disbelief, and denial. From what Worden (1982) says, the first task of mourning is for the bereaved person to accept the reality of the loss. This task is not dissimilar to those identified by Parkes and Weiss (1972), who believe that the bereaved person needs to recognise and accept the loss on two levels, intellectually and emotionally, in order to move to recovery. For Worden (1982), the bereaved person needs to 'come full face with the reality that the person is dead' (p. 11) and that reunion on earth is not possible. Worden also believes that those who are unable to accept the loss will become fixated at the stage of denial. This means staying at the stage where they continue to believe the loss has not taken place and would thus be seen as an abnormal response or maladaptive behaviour as it is often referred to. The concept of abnormal grief is discussed later on in this chapter. Grieving is a very sensitive period in a bereaved person's life and to hear someone say that one has to accept the reality of the loss (although true) can in itself be more traumatic for that person. For practitioners, therefore, it is not about informing what the state of affairs is or should be, but instead, they should demonstrate empathic understanding of the bereaved person's lived experience. Exercise 7 attempts to integrate the notion of accepting the reality of the loss with self-awareness.

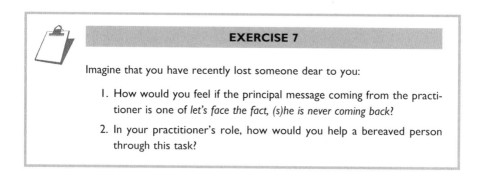

EXERCISE 7

Imagine that you have recently lost someone dear to you:

1. How would you feel if the principal message coming from the practitioner is one of *let's face the fact, (s)he is never coming back?*

2. In your practitioner's role, how would you help a bereaved person through this task?

It is beyond the scope of this chapter to offer a structured plan in relation to helping someone to work through Worden's (1982) task one. However, one of the guiding principles should be an awareness of how one might feel, think, and behave when faced with a loss. Self-knowledge can then be used to structure a plan based on sensitivity and empathic understanding in order to help the bereaved person.

Task two: To experience the pain of grief

During the normal course of grieving, the bereaved person will experience emotional as well as physical pain. However, the intensity of this pain varies from individual to individual depending on the depth of closeness or attachment with the dead person. Worden warns that society may play a part in making this task difficult with a message that 'You don't need to grieve'. The implication is that bereaved individuals may take this on board, thus denying themselves the opportunity to experience their true feelings. This begs the following questions. *How realistic is it to expect someone who has experienced the loss of a loved one not to feel pain? Why do we feel the need to say don't cry or don't be sad when faced with someone who has incurred a loss?* Perhaps Exercise 8 can shed some light on this behaviour.

EXERCISE 8

Explore some of the reasons why we may ask a bereaved person not to cry.

Whatever rationale one can offer from Exercise 8, the underpinning sentiment is that in most instances the tendency to say these things rests with our own feeling of discomfort in the presence of a bereaved person and we try our hardest to distract their feelings of loss. Gorer (1965) is quoted to have said, 'Giving way to grief is stigmatized as morbid, unhealthy, demoralizing. The proper action of a friend and well-wisher is felt to be distraction of a mourner from his or her grief' (Worden, 1982, p. 13). Perhaps, this is more to do with our own weaknesses of not knowing what to say when faced with someone who is grieving. This is reflected in a personal encounter with a colleague of mine whose death was imminent as a result of a terminal illness. Twelve years on I still remember these words. *Once word got round that I was dying of cancer, some people I have known since I was a child do their utmost to avoid contact with me even to the point of deliberately crossing the road to walk on the other side. It was as if I have a contagious disease* (Personal Communication). In truth, it was not so much that his friends believed that he had a contagious disease but more on the lines of *I don't really know what to say to you.* Exercise 9 encourages analytical thinking and self-awareness.

EXERCISE 9

As with Exercise 7, imagine that you have recently lost someone dear to you:
How would you wish friends, colleagues, or health care practitioners to behave towards you?
What might you do to avoid experiencing the pain of grief?

According to Worden (1982), in their attempt to cope with their loss, some people may try to find a 'geographical cure' instead of experiencing the pain of grief. One such example could be moving to a different location and making a fresh start. However, geographical cure should not be seen as the solution because it does not resolve issues but could even aggravate the problem.

Task three: To adjust to an environment in which the deceased is missing

Adjusting to the new environment depends on the extent to which the bereaved person has to change. According to Worden, this depends on the type of relationship individuals have had with the deceased.

For many widows it takes a considerable period of time to realize what it is like to live without their husbands. This realization often begins to emerge around three months after the loss and involves coming to terms with living alone, raising children alone, facing an empty house, and managing finances alone.

(Worden, 1982, p. 14)

The implication that the exact nature of the adjustment becomes visible only after the loss means that it can aggravate the existing pain. However, the necessity to make adjustment can force the bereaved person to acquire new skills in dealing with the new and uncharted territory.

Task four: To withdraw emotional energy and reinvest it in another relationship

For Worden (1982), withdrawing emotional energy and reinvesting it in another relationship should not be perceived as 'dishonoring the memory of the deceased' (p. 15). People are frightened to enter into a new relationship for a variety of reasons. You may wish to explore the notion of reinvesting emotional energy into another relationship from your own perspective (see Exercise 10).

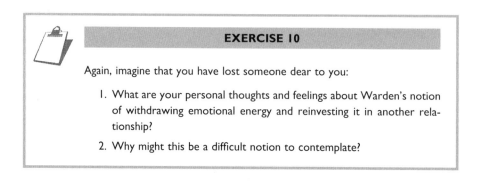

EXERCISE 10

Again, imagine that you have lost someone dear to you:

1. What are your personal thoughts and feelings about Warden's notion of withdrawing emotional energy and reinvesting it in another relationship?

2. Why might this be a difficult notion to contemplate?

There are numerous reasons why individuals who are grieving may not wish to even contemplate the idea of a new relationship after the loss of their loved one. Some of these are highlighted in Appendix 4.

In summary, it could be said that grief is a natural process and that faced with the loss of a loved one people will undergo a succession of experiences and provided there is no complication, will reach a period when they are able to make the necessary changes in either their behaviour and/or environment in response to the new demand created by the loss. Bowlby (1980), Parkes (1972), Kübler-Ross (1969), and Worden (1982) have all suggested what they believe grieving and the task of mourning involve. Similarities exist, the most obvious one being the normal or natural process that follows loss of a loved one. Although most of what has been said relates to death, the notion of grieving can be translated to any loss. The principal sentiment underpinning care is that people should be encouraged to engage with their feeling and thinking and only then are they able to adjust to their new situation. However, the question is, *when does grief become abnormal?* An attempt is made to offer some answers in the ensuing section.

Complicated and abnormal grief

Reflecting on Engel's (1961) sentiment (expressed earlier in the chapter), parallels can be drawn between illness and the process of grief with all its demands made on an individual following the loss of a loved one. However, not all illnesses are referred to health care professionals, for example, we don't all rush to our doctors at the first sign of flu. We are only inclined to seek medical help if all efforts in combating our flu prove fruitless. The same could be said for grieving. We may only seek professional help if we are unable to deal with our loss and our response is such that our situation is aggravated. Moreover, we would seek medical permission via a sick certificate to take a break from work. These in themselves are not sufficient to label grief as abnormal or complicated. There is no doubt that the experience of grief can result in maladapted behaviour. Exercise 11 provides an opportunity to explore the notion of abnormal grief.

EXERCISE 11

1. When does grieving become maladaptive?
2. Reflect on each of the theories presented above and identify some of the factors that could make the grieving process complicated and hence maladaptive.

Grief can be seen as a maladaptive response to loss when, for example, an individual is not able to move satisfactorily through the stages of the grieving process. Abnormal grief[4] responses to a loss can take various forms and these include delayed or prolonged grief (sometimes referred to as pathological or morbid grief reaction). Delayed grief[5] suggests that an individual does not show the experience of the emotion of pain usually associated with the loss object at the time of the loss. Moreover, individuals may remain in such a state until an external or internal trigger rekindles the initial response to that loss. By contrast, prolonged grief implies that an individual becomes preoccupied with the loss object for a number of years after the event. Appendix 5 offers some examples that could hinder the grieving process, thus leading to maladaptive behaviour. These could serve as topics for in depth discussions.

Recognising and managing the impact of loss in self and others

Worden (2003) states that knowledge about the tasks of grieving is only part of the equation in helping bereaved people. Another crucial element is understanding what he calls 'the *Mediators of Mourning*' (Worden, 2003, p. 38) and these are knowing who the dead person was, the nature of the attachment, mode of death, historical antecedents, personality variables, social variables, and concurrent stresses. It is not the intension here to discuss these mediators in detail as Worden (2003)[6] has done this with excellent clarity. However, Exercise 12 aims to generate some discussions.

EXERCISE 12

Discuss with one or two of your colleagues how an understanding of who the person was, the nature of the attachment, mode of death, historical antecedents (an individual's past experience of grieving), personality variables, social variables, and concurrent stresses contribute to the effectiveness of caring for the bereaved person. As with most of the exercises in this chapter, self-awareness could be used as a tool to help understanding the lived experience of the bereaved person.

The above exercises should give you a reasonable idea of the role these mediators play in relation to an individual's lived experience of loss. The belief is that if you are able to sense it and feel it from your own personal perspective you may develop a greater level of empathy with the bereaved person. The implication is that your level of self-awareness will dictate your effectiveness as a health care practitioner. For example, if I were the bereaved person, it would give me a greater sense of comfort to know that the person who is designated to support me has a good understanding of my situation. I might see that person as a really caring person for making the effort to find out as much of what there is to know about my circumstances.

The principles of engaging with the bereaved person

Before considering some of the principles of engagement it needs to be stressed that it is not intended here to give specific instructions in how you should help or what type of therapeutic interventions you should adopt in helping a bereaved person. Although my individual experience in dealing with mental health problems spans over a period of 30 years, I am not a trained counsellor nor am I a therapist, and it would be wrong to portray myself as such. However, reflecting on my clinical and educational experience over that period of time

I have come to believe health care practitioners need to possess some special attributes in order to fully engage with patients, and this sentiment is captured in the following quote.

> We know that if the therapist holds within himself attitudes of deep respect and full acceptance for this client as he is, and similar attitudes toward the client's potentialities for dealing with himself and his situations; if these attitudes are suffused with sufficient warmth, which transforms them into the most profound type of liking or affection for the core of the person; and if a level of communication is reached so that the client can begin to perceive that the therapist understands the feelings he is experiencing and accepts him at the full depth of that understanding, then we may be sure that the process [of helping] is already initiated.
>
> (Rogers, 1967, pp. 74–75)[7]

Reflecting on this sentiment, it becomes clear that the prerequisite for helping a bereaved person or anyone who feels a sense of loss for that matter, is the practitioner's ability to initiate, sustain, and terminate a relationship based on deep respect and full acceptance for that person. Moreover, these would contribute to a safe relationship where the client/patient would feel no inhibition in disclosing their thinking, feeling, and action. Parkes, Relf, and Couldrick (1996) state that in aiming to convey respect we need to believe that the person is worthwhile, unique, and valuable. Exercise 13 may help to explore the notion of respect.

EXERCISE 13

Identify a person whom you feel shows you respect. What does he or she say that makes you feel respected?

Below are some of the ways one can show respect for others.

- Recognise and accept people for whom they are.
- Listening in a non-judgemental way.
- Not interrupting when they are talking.
- Take the life position of 'I'm okay you're okay' (Harris, 1973).

Acceptance is closely linked with respect and according to Rogers (1967) is a 'warm regard for him as a person of unconditional self-worth – of value no matter what his condition, his behaviour, or his feelings' (p. 34). The implication is that both respect and acceptance are highly important elements in a helping relationship. Moreover, individuality and sensitivity are also important. Underpinned by respect and acceptance, one of the principles of engaging with a bereaved person is that he or she should be treated as a unique individual with unique needs because as Parkes and Weiss (1983) state, the 'forms of intervention which are appropriate for one type of bereavement may be useless or even harmful in another' (p. 227). This stresses the importance of getting to know the person as well as one possibly can. Exercise 14 may help in the process of getting to know the patient.

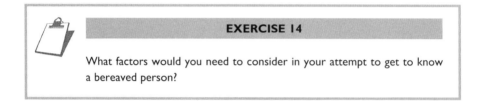

EXERCISE 14

What factors would you need to consider in your attempt to get to know a bereaved person?

The answers to the Exercise 14 may be found in Worden's (2003) mediators of mourning. However, one would suggest that looking at one's own reaction to loss might contribute greatly to one's effectiveness as a practitioner. For example, how do you deal with your own loss? What effect do you think losing someone or something may have on a person? Exercise 15 is structured to help facilitate this process.

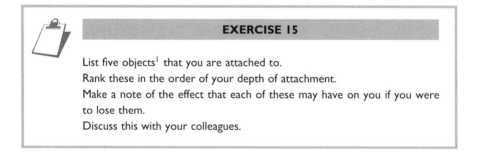

EXERCISE 15

List five objects[1] that you are attached to.
Rank these in the order of your depth of attachment.
Make a note of the effect that each of these may have on you if you were to lose them.
Discuss this with your colleagues.

In considering loss from a self-perspective we may come to realise our strengths and weaknesses in dealing with people who are bereaved. Moreover, Worden (2003) states, 'there is nothing like looking at a significant loss in one's own life to bring home the reality of the grief process' (p. 175). Exploring one's own personal history of loss may also help in generating a greater sense of awareness of other people's loss. Exercise 16 relates to one's personal history of loss as well as knowledge, skills, and attitudes.

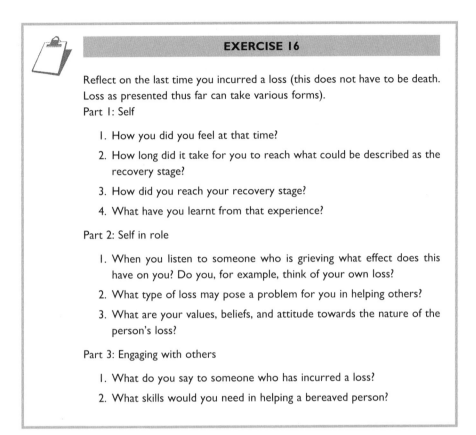

EXERCISE 16

Reflect on the last time you incurred a loss (this does not have to be death. Loss as presented thus far can take various forms).

Part 1: Self

1. How you did you feel at that time?

2. How long did it take for you to reach what could be described as the recovery stage?

3. How did you reach your recovery stage?

4. What have you learnt from that experience?

Part 2: Self in role

1. When you listen to someone who is grieving what effect does this have on you? Do you, for example, think of your own loss?

2. What type of loss may pose a problem for you in helping others?

3. What are your values, beliefs, and attitude towards the nature of the person's loss?

Part 3: Engaging with others

1. What do you say to someone who has incurred a loss?

2. What skills would you need in helping a bereaved person?

One of the aims of Exercise 16 is to encourage self-awareness in the context of loss and grief. The underlying principle is that self-knowledge increases practitioners' effectiveness. The whole emphasis therefore is upon translating this knowledge to clinical practice. Numerous issues would emerge from Exercise 16, and some of these could be used as classroom discussion in an attempt to further development.

Summary

Grief is described as one of the most complex of human emotions experienced as a result of loss of an object of attachment. However, the object needs to be significant in order to have an impact on an individual. In theory, the depth of attachment is said to determine the extent of the disturbance and by definition loss creates a sense of *emptiness*, which requires *adjustment* on the part of the individual. Adjustment in this context does not mean a *happy ending* but simply that individuals make the *best of a bad situation*. Coping therefore can be both adaptive and maladaptive as in the form of persistent denial or aggression. Denial and anger are two of the initial stages displayed in response to loss. A number of theorists believe that grieving follows a natural process that the bereaved person goes through. However, for some individuals this journey can be problematic in that they could be fixated at any one of the stages thus requiring input from health care professionals. The principal theme throughout this chapter in the context of loss and grief emphasises self-awareness on the part of the practitioner. The underpinning belief is that self-awareness could contribute greatly to a competent practitioner.

References

Bowlby, J. (1973). *Attachment and Loss Vol. II. Separation Anxiety and Anger*. London: The Hogarth Press and The Institute of Psycho-Analysis.

Bowlby, J. (1980). *Attachment and Loss: Loss, Sadness and Depression*. London: The Hogarth Press and The Institute of Psycho-Analysis.

Bowlby, J. (1982). *Attachment and Loss Vol. I Attachment*. London: The Hogarth Press and The Institute of Psycho-Analysis.

Cassidy, J. (1999). The nature of the child's ties. In J. Cassidy and P. R. Shaver (eds.), *Handbook of Attachment* (pp. 3–20). New York and London: The Guildford Press.

Down-Wamboldt, B. and Tamlyn, D. (1997). An international survey of death education trend in faculties of nursing and medicine. *Death Studies*, 21, 177–188.

Engel, G. L. (1961). Is grief a disease? A challenge for medical research. *Psychosomatic Medicine*, 23, 18–22.

Gorer, G. (1965). *Death, Grief and Mourning*. New York: Doubleday.

Harris, T. A. (1973). *I'm OK-You're OK*. London and Sydney: Pan Books.

Holmes, J (1993). *John Bowlby & Attachment Theory*. London and New York: Routledge.

Horowitz, M. J., Wilner, N., Marmar, C., and Krupnick, J. (1980). Pathological grief and the activation of latent self-images. *The American Journal of Psychiatry*, 137, 1157–1162.

Hsu, M. T., Tseng, Y. F., Banks, J. M., and Kuo, L. L. (2004). Interpretations of stillbirth. *Journal of Advanced Nursing*, 47(4), 408–416.

Kastenbaum, R. (2000). *The Psychology of Death*. London: Free Association Book Ltd.

Kobak, R. (1999). The emotional dynamics of disruptions in attachment relationships: implications for theory, research, and clinical intervention. In J. Cassidy and P. R. Shaver (eds.), *Handbook of Attachment* (pp. 21–43). New York and London: The Guildford Press.

Kübler-Ross, E. (1969). *On Death and Dying*. New York: Macmillan.

Parkes, C. M. (1971). Psychosocial transitions: a field for study. *Social Science and Medicine*, 5(2), 101–114.

Parkes, C. M. (1972). *Bereavement: Studies of Grief in Adult Life*. New York: International Universities Press.

Parkes, C. M. (1982). Attachment and the prevention of mental disorders. In C. M. Parkes and J. Hinde (eds.), *The Place of Attachment and Human Behaviors* (pp. 295–310). New York: Basic Books.

Parkes, C. M. (1996). *Bereavement: Studies of Grief in Adult Life*. London and New York: Routledge.

Parkes, C. M. and Weiss, R. S. (1983). *Recovery from Bereavement*. New York: Basic Books, Inc., Publishers.

Parkes, C. M., Relf, M., and Couldrick, A. (1996). *Counselling in Terminal Care and Bereavement*. Leicester: BPS Books.

Payne, S. and Horn, S. (1999). *Loss and Bereavement*. Buckingham and Philadelphia: Open University Press.

Prior, L. (1989). *The Social Organisation of Death: Medical Discourse and Social Practices in Belfast*. London: MacMillan.

Rando, T. A. (2000). The six dimensions of anticipatory mourning. In T. A. Rando (ed.), *Clinical Dimensions of Anticipatory Mourning: Theory and Practice in Working with the Dying, Their Loved Ones, and Their Caregivers* (pp. 51–101). Champaign, IL: Research Press.

Richards, A. (1984). *Sigmund Freud: On Metapsychology*. England: Penguin Books.

Rogers, C. R. (1967). *On Becoming a Person: A Therapist's View of Psychotherapy*. London: Constable.

Worden, W. J. (1982). *Grief Counselling and Grief Therapy*. London and New York: Tavistock Publications.

Worden, W. J. (2003). *Grief Counselling and Grief Therapy: A Handbook for the Mental Health Practitioner*. Hove and New York: Brunner-Routledge.

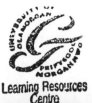

Anger, Aggression, and Self-Awareness

Dev M. Rungapadiachy

OBJECTIVES

After reading this chapter you should be able to

- Discuss the concepts of anger and aggression.

- Demonstrate your understanding of anger and aggression in self and others.

- Manage anger and aggression in self and others through self-awareness.

Introduction

Anger is said to be a natural and powerful emotion. This implies that it is okay to feel angry. However, if not channelled appropriately, anger can have a negative effect on both self and others. One could argue that the negative display of anger behaviour stems from what could be seen as people's lack of understanding of feelings that is further aggravated by their inability to express them in socially acceptable ways. In simple term, anger is something that most of us do not manage as well as we should do. This means that anger controls us and in turn we use it to control others. For health care practitioners, however, anger management is a prerequisite for effective health care delivery. This chapter focuses on some of the theories of anger and aggression. Emphasis is on practitioners' use of self-awareness through a variety of structured exercises in an attempt to increase self-knowledge that is crucial to effectively engaging with patients.

Anger and aggression defined

Anger can be described as an emotion that is often accompanied by thoughts of attacking. According to Berkowitz (1993a), anger refers to an internal drive state that impels an aggressive behaviour. Anger does not directly instigate aggression but only accompanies the inclination to attack a target. This means that individuals may sometimes try to hurt others more or less impulsively and without being consciously aware of themselves as angry. This lack of self-awareness therefore suggests that sometimes we may not always recognise our display of anger behaviour. Exercise 1 encourages reflection with the aim of increasing one's self-awareness in relation to anger.

EXERCISE I

Recall a time when you may not have been aware of your anger.

Aggression is described as 'a response that delivers noxious stimuli to another organism' (Buss, 1961, p. 1). However, Geen (2001) argues that aggression is not as simple as a behavioural definition would indicate. This means that other factors must be taken into account, for example, intent to harm and the motivation of the victim. It seems that for a specific behaviour to be seen as aggressive *there needs to be a clear intent of wanting to cause harm to others thus ruling out accidental acts where one person harms another*. Aggressive behaviour therefore has to be goal directed, and the goal needs to indicate a clear intent to cause harm. Baron and Richardson (1994) posit that aggression is any form of behaviour that is directed towards the goal of harming another human being who is motivated to avoid such treatment. This definition does not take into account the fact that in some situations victims may not be able to take evasive action either because of their inability to do so or because they may feel that avoiding actions may aggravate their situation. Another argument is that if victims attempt to defend themselves would they too be seen as aggressive? The answer may be 'yes', and this relates to the notion of instrumental aggression (discussed later in this chapter). Defining aggression can be problematic; however, what seems clear is that the levels of aggression, its target, and context will decide the extent to which aggression is acceptable or not. For example, aggression in a boxing ring would be considered normal and therefore acceptable. By comparison, aggression in a classroom setting is not seen as normal and hence not acceptable. Anderson and Bushman summarise their notion of accidental aggression, as

> accidental harm is not aggressive because it is not intended. Harm that is an incidental by-product of helpful actions is also not aggressive, because the harm-doer believes that the target is not motivated to avoid the action (e.g., pain experienced during a dental procedure). Similarly, the pain administered in sexual masochism is not aggressive because the victim is not motivated to avoid it – indeed, the pain is actively solicited in service of a higher goal.

(Anderson & Bushman, 2002, p. 28)

This begs the question, *is mercy killing an aggressive act?* This last question can serve as a topic for discussion. Based on Anderson and Bushman's explanation mercy killing may not be seen as an aggressive act; however, according to British law mercy killing is considered to be an act of aggression.

Other words closely linked with anger and aggression are hostility, rage, and hate. Berkowitz (1993a) defines hostility as 'a negative attitude towards one or more people that is reflected in a decidedly unfavourable judgement of the target' (p. 21). For example, clearly showing a dislike for someone would be perceived as being hostile towards that person. Hostility is not perceived as normal because we don't all have negative feelings towards others. Moreover, the negative attitude a hostile individual holds is usually followed by a desire for the target to suffer in some way. Hence, hostile aggression suggests that the person derives some element of pleasure in harming or seeking to harm others.

Wiener (1998) believes that anger and rage are linked affects. Affects are described as instinctive components of human behaviour that are common to all individuals. According to Kernberg (1995), affects 'emerge in the earliest stages of development and are gradually organized, as part of early object relations, into gratifying, rewarding, pleasurable affects or libido as an overarching drive, and painful, aversive, negative affects that, in turn, are organised into aggression as an overarching drive' (Akhter, Kramer, & Parens, 1995, p. 57). An object relation suggests that the primary relationship of an individual starts with mother and infant interaction and this together with intrapersonal and interpersonal experiences (see Chapter 7) form the basis for the development of the child's identity. Moreover, how one interprets this relationship dictates future relationships with others. For example, pleasurable experience may lead to positive behaviour, whereas painful experience may result in aggression. In terms of psychic functioning, anger is different from rage. For example, one could argue that anger is aroused when a desired goal is frustrated. 'As a way of overcoming obstacles, anger is usually conscious, ego-related, has a cognitive component and is up to a point controllable' (Wiener, 1998, p. 497). Moreover, anger is not destructive. Rage, on the other hand, is described as a primitive affect that evolves from the unconscious. 'It is unpredictable, unbounded and can feel exceedingly dangerous' (Wiener, 1998, p. 498). The source of rage is believed to be shame. For example, Dutton, Van Ginkle, and Starzomski (1995) found that recalled shaming action by parents were related to adult abusiveness displayed through a variety of behaviour leaving children feeling they were being punished for who they were and not for what they did. Moreover, Dutton (1999) states that shame converts instantly to rage in what is coined as the 'shame-rage spiral'. For example, shame leads to rage, which leads to more shame, and in turn leads to more rage (Wiener, 1998). The implication is that in an attempt to protect oneself 'from what feels subjectively like looming annihilation' the individual exhibits rage behaviour (Dutton, 1999, p. 436).

According to Yanay (2002), hate is an intense emotion. Unlike anger, hate is seen as undesirable, and when displayed it is unacceptable. However, Lazar (2003) posits that hatred is seen as an aggressive drive pushing the psychic apparatus from its very beginning alongside the sexual drive. According to

Freud (1915), hatred is an ego response, for example, 'the ego hates, abhors, and pursues with intent to destroy all objects which are a source of unpleasurable feeling for it' (p. 138). The implication is that hate is an ego attitude with the intent of destructive aggression. Although hate and rage are bound together there is no simple relationship between them (Blum, 1995). For example, hate may be present without rage, but rage is always associated with hate. Exercise 2 is meant to serve as an introduction to the various forms of aggression.

EXERCISE 2

Identify some of the forms of aggression that you are aware of and/or that you have engaged in.

Forms of aggression

Reflecting on the brainstorming words highlighted in Appendix 6, perhaps it would be fair to say that most of us would have engaged in at least one of these behaviours in one way or another. The following anecdotal account was personally witnessed.

The relationship between the boss (Mr. D) and his employee (Miss. C) could be described as volatile. Mr. D always seems to be antagonistic and dehumanising towards Miss. C who, in her attempt to avoid confrontation, made her trips to the toilet to coincide with Mr. D's entrance to the unit. Unaware of the effect of his behaviour on Miss. C, Mr. D felt that he needed to establish the reason why Miss. C always disappeared at his mere presence. One occasion when Miss C was about to make her way to the toilet, Mr. D, in front of an audience, called her and said, 'Miss. C why is it that every time I come here you disappear to the toilet?' After a long pause, Miss C replied, 'well to tell you the truth Mr. D every time I see your face I feel I want to shit'.

It was clear from her behaviour that Miss. C did not want to confront the situation but instead felt comfortable in her covert expression of her anger. Mr. D had different ideas. He thought he had the upper hand over Miss. C and the worse of it was he thought he would make an example of Miss. C through a public confrontation. Mr. D's behaviour could also be seen as aggressive given that he planned to make Miss C look foolish in the presence of others. From an observer's perspective one can't help but to wonder *how does one recover face from Miss C's response?*

Geen's (2001) offers a working definition of aggression that suggests the delivery of an aversive stimulus from one person to another, with the intent to harm and with the expectation of causing such harm, when the other person is motivated to escape or avoid the stimulus. From this perspective therefore, aggression can range from spreading vicious gossip with the aim of ruining

Table 5.1 Shows a summary of the categories of aggressive behaviour

Type of aggression	Explanation	Example
Physical-active-direct	An act of physical assault carried out by the perpetrator against the victim	Bart punches Lisa
Physical-active-indirect	Using a third party to carry out an assault on someone	Homer hires Bart to beat up Lisa
Physical-passive-direct	A non-violent act that is aimed at preventing others to reach their goal	Bart locks Homer up in the toilet
Physical-passive-indirect	Non-involvement that leads to some form of disruption	Homer refuses to move during a sit in at the plant
Verbal-active-direct	Making a derogatory remark towards another person	Bart swears at Lisa
Verbal-active-indirect	Making derogatory remarks about person A to person B	Bart expresses negative attitude about Lisa to Marje
Verbal-passive-direct	Remaining silent when questioned	Homer refuses to respond to Bart
Verbal-passive-indirect	Not speaking up on behalf of someone else when he or she is unfairly criticised.	Homer says nothing when Bart criticises Lisa

Based on the idea of Baron, R. A. and Richardson, D. (1994). *Human Aggression* (p. 10). New York: Plenum.

someone's life to physically destroying someone's property. According to Baron and Richardson (1994), the variety of specific aggressive acts available to human beings is virtually endless. Moreover, a conceptual framework proposed by Buss (1961) shows three dimensions to aggression. These are physical-verbal, active-passive, and direct-indirect (see Table 5.1).

Affective and instrumental aggression

There are principally two kinds of aggression and these are affective and instrumental. Affective aggression (also referred to as emotional aggression) can be described as violent acts initiated by intense anger. For example, we feel angry at being provoked, and we display aggressive behaviour in an attempt to harm the person. Affective aggression tends to be displayed spontaneously and is not seen as entirely premeditated. However, it is not uncommon for an individual to display a delayed response to affective aggression. Instrumental aggression can be described as violent acts on others with the intent to harm but without necessarily feeling any malice towards them. For example, if we are being attacked and our only option is to retaliate with violence this would be interpreted as instrumental aggression. Instrumental aggression is different to hostile aggression in that the latter derives pleasure in making the victim suffer. Instrumental aggression is simply a means to an end as in *we do what we feel we have to.*

Anger profile

One of the simplest of exercises that can help to create an anger profile is a personal reflection that contributes to raising one's self-awareness (see Exercise 3).

EXERCISE 3

Reflect on your own behaviour (feeling, thinking, and actions) and ask yourself the following questions.

1. What makes me angry?
2. How do I behave when I am angry?
3. What are the consequences of my angry behaviour?

Questions from Exercise 3 are based on the notions of antecedents, behaviour, and consequences. An antecedent is any event that leads to an action. Antecedent could also be seen as a stimulus. Behaviour means any action taken in response to the antecedent. Consequence is described as the outcome of an action. You could extend your profile by working with the questionnaire from Table 5.2. The questionnaire is only intended to raise self-awareness in relation to your thinking, feeling, and action regarding your experience of anger. Its validity is only restricted for that purpose. Issues for discussion can be found in Table 5.3. Each question relates to the corresponding question in Table 5.2. For example, if you have answered 'yes' to question 1 (I show my anger when I am provoked), then what you would need to be asking yourself is *how do I show my anger and what is it that other people have to do to provoke me?* Of course, there is an assumption here that the answer to each question in Table 5.2 is true. This may not necessarily be the case, however, it should help to generate discussions.

EXERCISE 4

Table 5.2 Anger and aggression questionnaire

	Statement	True	False
1.	I show my anger when I am provoked		
2.	If someone hits me I will defend myself even if this means hurting him or her		
3.	I can't stand the sight of some people		
4.	In the past I have threatened physical violence to others		

<table>
<tr><td colspan="2" align="center">**EXERCISE 4**</td></tr>
<tr><td>5.</td><td>I have been physically aggressive to at least one person</td></tr>
<tr><td>6.</td><td>I have a short fuse and I get angry very easily</td></tr>
<tr><td>7.</td><td>I bear feelings of resentment (grudge) when I am offended. I have difficulty in forgiving people who have hurt me</td></tr>
<tr><td>8.</td><td>I have said things to others that I have regretted later</td></tr>
<tr><td>9.</td><td>When I get angry, I stay angry for hours</td></tr>
<tr><td>10.</td><td>I have been angry to the point of losing control</td></tr>
<tr><td>11.</td><td>Those who know me can usually tell when I am angry</td></tr>
<tr><td>12.</td><td>I usually feel guilty after having expressed my anger</td></tr>
<tr><td>13.</td><td>I am secretly quite critical of others</td></tr>
<tr><td>14.</td><td>I get angry when someone lets me down</td></tr>
<tr><td>15.</td><td>I get angry when people are unfair to me or to others</td></tr>
<tr><td>16.</td><td>I get angry when things get in my way</td></tr>
<tr><td>17.</td><td>I get angry when I have to work with people I perceive as incompetent</td></tr>
<tr><td>18.</td><td>In an argument I always want to win</td></tr>
<tr><td>19.</td><td>I analyse events that make me angry</td></tr>
<tr><td>20.</td><td>I feel uncomfortable in the presence of someone who is angry</td></tr>
</table>

Table 5.3 Issues for discussion

Statement	Issues for discussion
1.	How do you show your anger when provoked and what does it take to provoke you?
2.	To what extent of physical violence are you prepared to engage in?
3.	Ever asked yourself why you can't stand the sight of someone's face. Given that this is the case how do you behave towards that person?

Statement	Issues for discussion
4.	To whom have you threatened physical violence and why? How can you justify yourself?
5.	Why were you physically aggressive in the past and what was the outcome?
6.	Why the short fuse?
7.	How does feeling resentment influence your thinking and action?
8.	What have you learnt from that experience?
9.	What do you do and how do you know that you are still angry?
10.	How aware are you when you are about to lose control?
11.	What cues can others pick up?
12.	You expressed your anger once and you feel guilty about it. Have you learnt from past behaviour? Or what have you learnt from it?
13.	Can you work out why you are critical of others? Are you as critical of yourself as you are of others? What's that about? For example, do people deserve your critique?
14.	Have you ever let anyone down?
15.	Have you always been fair?
16.	Have you ever been in other people's way?
17.	Would you consider yourself perfect? Have you ever felt incompetent?
18.	What is the need to win related to?
19.	What conclusion have you come up with?
20.	Why might you feel uncomfortable in the presence of someone who is angry?

Both Tables 5.2 and 5.3 (Exercise 4) should help to create a profile of anger based on the following.

■ Frequency of anger: How often do I feel angry?

■ Duration of anger: How long does each experience of my anger last?

■ Magnitude: What is the extent of my anger?

■ Mode of expression: How do I express anger? For example, *do I keep it in or do I let rip*?

■ Would this behaviour be acceptable or unacceptable and/or adaptive or maladaptive? (The notions of adaptive and maladaptive are explained briefly in Chapter 2.)

Causes of aggression

According to Krahé (2001), whether or not an individual will react with an aggressive response to an aversive stimulation depends to a high degree on how the stimulation is interpreted by the recipient. The implication is that frustrations are much more likely to elicit anger behaviour when interpreted as deliberate. According to Todorov and Bargh (2002), people who are repeatedly exposed to stimuli related to aggression can develop chronically accessible knowledge structures, which would automatically affect the interpretation of new aggression-related events. This means that our perception of aggression depends on who we are and how we have come to be who we are. A further implication is that past experience is a significant factor in one's perception of aggression. Therefore, a much more effective way to establish some of the causes of aggression is to brainstorm some ideas among colleagues (see Exercise 5).

EXERCISE 5

This exercise is an extension of 'what makes me angry'. Here you could brainstorm what makes people angry by using self as a source of knowledge.

Emerging issues could include injustice, self-defence, defence of one's property, stress and anxiety, protecting others, frustration, feeling fobbed off, and discrimination.

Causes of aggression in health care settings

Violence in health care settings is described as a pervasive epidemic that constitutes an occupational hazard (Rippon, 2000). It would be wrong to believe that aggression in health care settings is confined solely to one group of health care professionals (that is, nurses) or areas such as mental health, and accident & emergency units (A&E). In fact, doctors, radiographers, and physiotherapists have all reported being assaulted (Winstanley & Whittington, 2004). Moreover, Whittington, Shuttleworth, and Hill (1996) showed that 90% of the reported assaults occurred outside the A&E units. In 1987, the Health Services Advisory Committee reported that by comparison staff in medical wards were more at risk than those on A&E units. Similarly, staff on surgical and orthopaedics wards were also at risk of assault. Some (Naish et al., 2002) argue that it is difficult to determine the true extent of the problem of aggression and violence caused by patients against primary care workers because much of what has been written is anecdotal or based on relatively small samples. There is a clear indication that the display of aggressive behaviour can be found in all health care settings. An interesting point, however, is that although aggressive behaviour may be widespread in all areas of health care this does not necessarily mean that all violence stems from patients or their relatives. Aggression against co-workers is as rampant as aggressive behaviour from patients or patients' relatives. For

Table 5.4 Some causes of aggression in health care setting

Physical illness	Psychotic illness where hallucination and delusion are acted upon	Drug or alcohol use	Lack of information
Stress, anxiety, and fear	Preventing patients from being discharged	Noisy environment	Lack of space
Interference from other patients	Confusion	Arguments over medication	Preventing patients from leaving the wards
Frustration	As a means of gaining staff's attention		

example, doctors were reported for being aggressive towards nurses (Farrell, 1999). Moreover, Farrell (2001) states that a major complaint of nurses is poor colleague relationships across a number of different work settings.

One of the most common antecedents of aggression in health care settings revolves round interpersonal factors. Kurlowitz (1990) found that patients often attribute interpersonal confrontations as an important cause for displaying aggressive behaviour. For example, patients are angered or annoyed by intrusive or frustrating behaviour of others. This can be from both patients and staff. However, some have gone so far as to suggest that staff sometimes subtly encourage patients' aggression by displacing their own feelings onto them (Dubin, 1989). Moreover, Gillig et al. (1998) found that verbal abuse of patients by staff was a major cause of physical aggression on one psychiatric unit. Similarly, Rungapadiachy (2003) found some nurses to be aggressive towards patients.

Another factor contributing to aggression and violence is patients' feeling of powerlessness. For example, Secker et al. (2004) found that patients' power-lessness to be a dominant theme for their aggressiveness. In this instance, the displayed aggression is perceived 'as a brief instance of self-empowerment' (p. 173). Some views of causality of aggression can be seen in Table 5.4.

Theories of anger and aggression

There are various theories of anger and aggression, and these rest principally within biological and psychological perspectives. Biological theories include at least three perspectives and these are ethology, socio-biology, and heredity and hormones. Psychological theories include psychoanalytical model, frustration–aggression hypothesis, cognitive models, learning theory, and social interactionist model.

Ethological model

The ethological model conceptualises aggression as an internal energy. One of the leading figures in this field is Lorenz (1966), who proposes that an organism continuously builds up aggressive energy. Lorenz argues that aggression originates from an innate fighting instinct that human beings have in common with other organisms. From this, Baron and Richardson (1994) presume that such an instinct develops during the long course of evolution because it serves three important functions.

1. Fighting disperses members of a species over a wide geographic area and in so doing ensuring maximal utilisation of available food resources.

2. Aggression helps to strengthen the genetic makeup of the species by guaranteeing that only the strongest and the most vigorous individuals will manage to reproduce.

3. The strongest animals are better able to protect and assure the survival of their offspring.

However, the display of aggression depends on two factors and these are as follows.

1. The amount of aggressive energy accumulated inside the organism at any one time.

2. The strength of external stimuli capable of triggering an aggressive response.

According to Krahé (2001), these two factors are inversely related. This means that the lower the energy level, the stronger the stimulus required to elicit an aggressive response. In simple terms, this person is described as having a long fuse. Similarly, the greater the amount of aggressive energy present, the weaker the stimulus that will help to release overt aggression. Such a person is said to have a short fuse. Moreover, Baron and Richardson (1994) add that if sufficient time has elapsed since the performance of the last aggressive act, such behaviour may occur in a spontaneous manner, in the total absence of releasing stimuli. The implication is that one does not necessarily need to have a stimulus to trigger an aggressive response. Lorenz posits that a low level of aggressive energy can be maintained if an individual were to participate in many minor, non-injurious aggressive actions regularly. For example, engaging in sports competitions would mean that levels of aggressive energy would be maintained below the critical threshold where violent outburst and other destructive behaviour would be kept in check.

Socio-biological model

The socio-biological model has its foundation in Darwin's (1859) theory of evolution, which is the 'origin of species'. Its basic principle is that in order to survive the organism has to be adaptive to its environment and only the strongest will survive. According to Krahé (2001), aggressive behaviour that is directed at fighting off attackers as well as rivals in mate selection is seen as adaptive in the sense of enhancing the reproduction success of the aggressor and in so doing they would ensure the continued success of future generations. Socio-biologists would argue that people will more likely contribute to the continued survival of those who share their genes by engaging in altruistic or self-sacrificing acts

(Baron & Richardson, 1994). For example, when food is scarce a mother will most likely feed her children rather than feed herself.

Heredity and hormonal explanations

The principal argument the heredity model holds is that aggressive behaviour is inherited. This means that aggression is passed on from parents to children. However, as pointed out by Krahé, 'most children are brought up by their biological parents, to whom they are genetically related, the effects of "nature" and "nurture" normally coincide in individual development' (p. 31). It becomes difficult therefore to say categorically that genes transmitted from parent to child are responsible for the child's aggressive behaviour. Adoption and twin studies can provide some indications as to the significance of hereditary influences. According to Geen (2001), the evidence from twin studies on the role of inherited biological factors in human aggression is mixed and inconclusive. However, Berkowitz (1993) states that research comparing monozygotic and dizygotic twins, which go back at least to the 1920s, has consistently demonstrated that a tendency to criminality may be heritable.

Testosterone, the principal androgenic (producing masculine characteristics) hormone is perhaps best known in aggression among non-human animals (Geen, 2001). For example, according to Archer (1988), one widespread mechanism that increases the readiness of male birds and mammals to fight during the mating seasons is the action of testosterone on areas of the brain controlling aggressive behaviour. The link between testosterone and aggression in birds was proposed by the 'challenge hypothesis' that states that there is a moderate rise in the levels of testosterone in order to support reproductive behaviour (Wingfield et al., 1990). Moreover, when males are challenged, 'in contexts that are relevant to reproduction, testosterone levels rise further. In turn, this facilitates aggression in the context of territory formation, dominance disputes, and mate-guarding' (Archer, 2006, p. 320). In humans, the picture is still mixed with some believing that testosterone is significant while others disclaim its contribution. However, reviewing the literature on testosterone–behaviour relationship, Archer (2006) proposes six hypotheses (see Table 5.5) to show how the 'challenge hypothesis' can be applied to human.

Psychoanalytical model

Freud (1920) believes that people's inner urges drive them towards theirs particular goals. This means that an individual is driven by two principal instincts. These are Eros, the instinct of life, and Thanatos, the instinct of death. On the death instinct Freud (1993) had this to say, 'the one set of instincts, which work essentially in silence, would be those which follow the aim of leading the living creature to death and therefore deserve to be called the *"death instincts"*; these would be directed outwards... and would manifest themselves as *destructive* or *aggressive* impulses' (p. 157). Moreover, *Thanatos* is 'at work in every living being and is striving to bring it to ruin and to reduce life to its original condition of inanimate matter' (Freud, 1930, p. 67). Freud posits that people's ultimate

Table 5.5 Archer's (2006) six applications of challenge hypoptheses

Number	Hypothesis
One	There is no increase in aggression at puberty
Two	1. Men respond to sexual arousal with increased testosterone
	2. Men respond to competition with increased testosterone
Three	Testosterone response to challenge increases aggression
Four	Testosterone levels are lower among paternal men
Five	Aggressive dominance is correlated with testosterone levels
Six	Testosterone is associated with alternative life history strategies[1]

wants are not the gratification of their basic biological needs for survival but instead they have a wish to die. However, *Eros* and *Thanatos* are antagonistic towards one another and are as a result in a state of constant conflict that can be resolved only by diverting the destructive force away from the person onto others. According to Aronson, Wilson, and Akert (1997), Freud's view on aggression can be characterised as a hydraulic theory. For example, water pressure builds up in a container and unless aggression is allowed to drain off, it will produce some sort of explosion. It is not the intension to offer a critique of psychoanalytical explanations of aggression or any of the models presented in this chapter for that matter. Whether the notion of life and death instincts makes sense or not is a matter of personal opinion in most cases as it would be difficult for research to validate those intrapersonal elements. However, it is not uncommon to hear people say, *I wish I was dead* when faced with life's problems. Perhaps one should not rush to discard the idea of life and death instincts.

Frustration–aggression model

The frustration–aggression hypothesis was first proposed by Dollard et al. (1939), and it states that frustration leads to aggression. Frustration is taken to mean an external condition that prevents a person from obtaining the pleasures he or she had expected to enjoy (Berkowitz, 1993). Dollard et al.'s (1939) original hypothesis was that the occurrence of aggression always presupposes the existence of frustration. Similarly, the existence of frustration always leads to some form of aggression. This was later revised by Miller (1941) to mean, 'frustration produces instigations to a number of different types of response, one of which is an instigation to some form of aggression' (p. 338). The implication is that aggression is one possible response to frustration. Miller (1941) argues that instigation to aggression may occupy any one of a number of positions in the hierarchy of instigations aroused by a specific situation that is frustrating. For example, if frustration leads to a number of responses such as lacking in confidence, hopelessness, highly motivated, angry, and rage, the intensity of each of these responses will dictate which response is exhibited. If rage is felt more than lacking in confidence when an individual is being frustrated then the exhibited behaviour will be that of rage. Similarly, if hopelessness is more intense then the predominant behaviour will be that of helplessness. Moreover, if the instigation to aggression is the strongest member of this hierarchy, then acts of aggression will be the first response to occur. Baron and Richardson (1994) conclude that frustration sometimes facilitates aggression. However, this would depend on numerous mediating factors. Four of these factors are highlighted below.

- **The magnitude of frustration experienced by the potential aggressors**: The implication is that the effect of frustration on aggression depends heavily on the extent to which one is frustrated. For example, a high level of frustration may lead to aggression in contrast to a low level that induces little or no aggression.

- **The presence of aggressive cues**: It is argued that people are much more likely to exhibit aggressive behaviour when exposed to aggressive cues. For example, Gustafson (1986) found that those participants who had previously watched a film that depicted a street gang fight were more aggressive than those who watched a film that showed a car race.

- **The extent to which thwarting is arbitrary or unexpected**: The argument here is that individuals who expect to feel frustrated will show a much lower level of frustration than those who did not expect frustration.

- **Emotional and cognitive process of the frustrated potential aggressor**: For aggression to occur, the frustration must be unpleasant enough to produce negative affect (Baron & Richardson, 1994). Moreover, if the frustration does not arouse negative feelings then aggression will not occur. A further factor that is implicated is thought (cognition). According to Berkowitz (1988), if frustration does produce an unpleasant emotional experience then an individual's cognitive processes will influence the actual behaviour. For example, if the negative affect is interpreted as fear then the exhibited behaviour will most likely be linked with the thought of escaping or avoidance. Similarly, if the experienced feeling is anger the exhibited behaviour will be a tendency to aggress.

Learning theories of aggression

There are two principal learning theories and these are behavioural and cognitive. Behaviourists see learning primarily as a function of the environment where people learn reflexively and/or respond purposefully in accordance with the prevailing situation. Behaviourists would argue that antecedents and consequences are the two main determinants of aggression, thus leading to two types of learning. For example, those who emphasise the significance of antecedents see aggression as a response to being classically conditioned. Moreover, where the nature of the consequence of aggressive behaviour dictates a behaviour, operant conditioning is said to be at play. Both classical and operant conditionings are discussed below. The cognitive explanation of learning by contrast emphasises the acquisition, organisation, coding, storing, and the retrieval of information through mental processing. Cognitivists would place aggressive behaviour very much with each individual instead of the environment. Aggression, therefore, is more a question of how one's environment is perceived by self. For example, the chances of the display of aggressive behaviour are likely to be greater when an individual perceives his or her environment to be hostile than when it is perceived as pleasant. However, even in a hostile environment it is possible for the ensuing behaviour not to be aggressive as in *fight* but could instead be evasive as in *flight*. In this instance, individuals would engage in some cognitive processes, thus appraising their chances of winning or losing.

Classical conditioning

Classical conditioning is said to take place when two stimuli are repeatedly paired until the presence of one evokes the expectation of the other. This was demonstrated in Pavlov's (1927) classic experiment where food, which has the property of eliciting saliva, was repeatedly paired with the sound of a bell as the dog was being fed. Pavlov found that when the bell was sounded without the presence of food the dog would continue to salivate. He concluded that the dog had associated the sound of the bell with food. In a similar process an individual can be classically conditioned to be aggressive. According to Baron and Richardson (1994), a stimulus may acquire aggressive meaning by being associated with positively reinforced aggression. Moreover, stimuli that are repeatedly associated with anger instigators may gradually acquire the capacity to elicit aggressive actions from individuals who have previously been frustrated. For example, the mere presence of police officers in riot gear may instigate an individual's aggressive behaviour. As can the wearing of a Manchester United football shirt in front of say Arsenal supporters. The principles of classical conditioning would also seem to underpin the notion of priming. Priming can be described as the presentation of prior ideas or sentiments that would serve to trigger a memory, thus making it more accessible. According to Berkowitz (1993), the main idea that underpins priming is that when people encounter a stimulus that has a particular meaning, other ideas are triggered that have much the same meaning. This means that the exposure to violent scenes 'may activate a complex set of associations that are related to aggressive ideas or emotions, thereby temporarily increasing the accessibility of aggressive thoughts, feelings, and scripts (including aggressive action tendencies)' (Anderson et al., 2003, p. 95).

Operant conditioning

Operant conditioning is based on Thorndike's (1932) concept of law of effect, which essentially states that if a particular behaviour is rewarded it will most likely recur, whereas a behaviour that is followed by discomfort will not. Operant conditioning is based on the idea that a behaviour is followed by a consequence, and the nature of the consequence influences an individual's tendency to repeat or not to repeat similar behaviour. Thorndike's theory was extended by Skinner (1971), who contends that learning an abnormal pattern of behaviour is not always acquired by the simple pairing of a stimulus with a response such as classical conditioning but by producing new responses under conditions of reinforcement that is contingent on what the person does. For example, if parents were to reward their children when the latter displays aggressive behaviour they will most likely repeat such behaviour. It becomes clear, therefore, that the consequences of aggressive behaviour will determine whether such behaviour is repeated or not. This points to the type of reinforcement, for example, positive, negative, and punishment.

Positive reinforcement and aggressive behaviour

According to Berkowitz (1993), some people who are prone to violence continue to be aggressive because they have been rewarded for such behaviour. The implication is that they have come to learn that it pays to be aggressive. Positive reinforcement of aggressive behaviour occurs when the behaviour is followed by the presentation of some sort of reward. The reward serves to increase the probability of the recurrence of aggressive response. However, according to Renfrew (1997), positive reinforcement of aggressive behaviour happens under the control of discriminative stimuli that are associated with the probable success. For example, it is unlikely that a *mugger* will attack people who look as though they can defend themselves.

Negative reinforcement and aggressive behaviour

According to Renfrew (1997), one of the basic principles of operant conditioning is negative reinforcement. The implication is that behaviours are reinforced or strengthened by removal (escape) or prevention of (avoidance) some aversive condition. Negative reinforcement can be described as the removal of an aversive stimulus as a consequence of a behaviour, thus increasing the probability of the occurrence of that particular behaviour. For example, if individuals come to realise that they are going to be attacked they may decide to attack first, thus avoiding the aversive stimulus. Renfrew (1997) states that negative reinforcement serves as an adaptive device in order to limit an organism's exposure to damaging conditions. 'Since the conditions involved in aggression, such as painful stimulation, are typically aversive, it should come as no surprise that negative reinforcement sometimes is the basis of learned aggression' (Renfrew, 1997, p. 128).

Punishment and aggressive behaviour

The phenomenon of punishment suggests that a painful stimulus is inflicted in an attempt to prevent the repetition of the corresponding activity. However, punishment only suppresses the behaviour but does not eradicate it. This implies that when punishment or the threat of it is removed the initial response may return. It is debatable whether punishment is an appropriate tool for the elimination of aggressive behaviour. According to Skinner (1953), the complex nature of punishment is such that it can generate more problems in an individual. For example, smacking a child for misbehaving may produce guilt, fear, and pain, and these may suppress the undesired behaviour. Moreover, if the child misbehaves again, the conditioned guilt, fear, and pain may reappear, thus *forcing* him or her to discontinue with the behaviour. However, the additional problems may be the child's experience of guilt and fear that can have serious implications. According to Gershoff (2002), psychologists and other professionals are divided on the question of whether the benefits of corporal punishment might outweigh any potential hazards. However, in her meta-analysis of 88 studies that examined the association between parental corporal punishment and children's behaviour, Gershoff (2002) concludes that the effect of corporal punishment has both positive and negative implications. Some of the areas are considered below.

- **Immediate compliance**: According to Gershoff (2002), the primary goal most parents have in administering corporal punishment is to stop children from misbehaving immediately. She cites the work of Newsom, Flavell, and Rincover (1983) to point out that corporal punishment did indeed result in short-term compliance on the part of the children under investigation.

- **Moral internalisation**: The notion of moral internalisation suggests that children take on the values and attitudes of society as though these are their own, provided, of course, that minimal parental discipline is used. Moreover, for moral internalisation to be effective parents would need to provide their children with choices and rationales for the desirable behaviour; otherwise, corporal punishment may be detrimental to children.

- **Aggression**: There are numerous literature that implicate punishment with children's aggressive behaviour. In fact as far back as 1960, Hoffman concluded that unqualified power assertion[2] techniques in the forms of direct commands, threats, deprivations, and physical force can have a detrimental effect on the child as these evoke oppositional behaviour as well as feelings of hostility towards parents. Moreover, Huesmann, Eron, and Dubow (2002, p. 187) posit that harsh punishment 'might be correlated with criminality because it stimulates antisocial behaviour or because aggressive children stimulate harsh punishment and aggressive children tend to become antisocial'.

- **Delinquent, criminal, and antisocial behaviour**: According to Gershoff (2002), decades of research have shown corporal punishment to be associated with criminal and antisocial behaviour.

- **Parent–child relationship**: The argument here is that if parents are to inflict corporal punishment on their children this could disrupt the parent–child relationship in that children will learn to fear parents. According to Bugentall and Goodnow (1998), 'when children focus on parent as a source of fear-inducing messages, they are less likely to integrate the parent's message into a full understanding of the disciplinary event' (p. 419), hence, children may adopt avoidance behaviour.

Social cognitive learning theory

Described as the most influential of all social learning theorists, Bandura (1973) felt that neither classical nor operant conditioning offers sufficient explanation of human behaviour. For example, people don't just react to a situation or that behaviour is solely dependent on reinforcement, and 'if reinforcement of operant behaviours provided the sole means of learning about the outcomes of firing a gun at another person, eating poisonous plants, jumping over a cliff or falling into a stormy sea, few people would live long' (Howe, 1980, p. 129). Moreover, neither classical nor operant conditioning would generate new behaviour. Relying on the concept of trial and error as one way of learning new behaviour would be a time-consuming process. According to Bandura (1986, p. 47), if one has to rely on one's own action to learn new behaviour 'the process of cognitive and social development would be greatly retarded, not to mention exceedingly tedious. The constraints of time, resources, and mobility impose severe limits on the situations and activities that can be directly explored. Without informative guidance, much of one's efforts would be expended on costly errors and needless toil.' Bandura subscribes to the belief that learning can take place through watching what others do. According to Howe (1980), one way is through watching other people behave, and in doing so an individual 'can acquire habits, skills, and knowledge without having to directly experience the consequences of every single action' (p. 129). Bandura (1973) firmly believes that cognitive processes are involved in behaviour and people act the way they do because they would have made some sort of interpretation of their situation. Moreover, social behaviour is widely regulated by verbal cues. For example, an individual's behaviour can be influenced by suggestion, requests, and commands. Bandura (1973) states that these cues often operate in subtle ways as, 'parents are quick to issue commands to their children, but they do not always see to it that their requests are heeded. Children are therefore inclined to ignore demands voiced in mild or moderate tones' (Bandura, 1973, p. 46). However, parents' aggressive demands or commands serve as cues that they will enforce compliance if their demands are not heeded. Bandura goes on to say that of the numerous cues that influence how people will behave at any given moment, none is more apparent or effective than the actions of others. For example, we applaud when others clap; we make our way to the buffet table as soon as we see others move. The implication is that behaviour is prompted and channelled by what Bandura (1973. p. 46) calls 'the power of example'.

Bandura (1973) argues that modelling plays an important role in the rapid contagion of aggression. This means that aggressive behaviour can be learned by observing an influential model behaving in an aggressive manner. In the classic study conducted by Bandura, Ross, and Ross (1961) social transmission of aggression through the power of example was clearly demonstrated. Children who were exposed to aggressive condition, for example, in the presence of the experimental model displaying aggressive behaviour towards a Bobo doll (a plastic inflated toy, decorated as a clown and weighted at the bottom so that it bounces back up when pushed or punched), showed a good deal of physical and verbal aggressive behaviour resembling that of the models. By contrast, children who were exposed to non-aggressive models and those who had no previous exposure to any models rarely performed such responses. Bandura, Ross, and Ross (1961) state, 'the fact, however, that subjects expressed their aggression in ways that clearly resembled the novel patterns exhibited by the models provides striking evidence for the occurrence of learning by imitation'

(p. 580). Interestingly, imitation of film-mediated models was found to be as significant as the real-life models. For example, 'subjects who viewed the real-life models and the film-mediated models do not differ from each other in total aggressiveness' (Bandura, Ross, & Ross, 1963, p. 7).

Social interaction theory

Social interaction is what Goffman (1967) calls the class of events that occurs during co-presence and by virtue of co-presence. The implication is that the mere presence of others has a tendency to influence the way an individual behaves. Social interaction is a dynamic, changing sequence of behaviour between individuals (or groups of individuals) who modify their actions and reactions due to the actions by their interaction partner(s). Social interactions are events where people attach meaning to a situation, interpret what others are meaning, and respond accordingly. According to Cahagan (1984), co-presence is a minimal kind of interaction that serves two specific functions: (a) people monitor and control their own behaviour and (b) they monitor the behaviour of others and adjust their own behaviour accordingly. Social interaction theory, therefore, would interpret aggressive behaviour as a form of social influence (Anderson & Bushman, 2002). This implies that person A would use aggressive behaviour to produce some change in person B's behaviour. A's behaviour is directed by what he or she expects to gain from that particular interaction. Anderson and Bushman (2002) believe that social interaction theory 'provides an excellent way to understand recent findings that aggression is often the result of threats to high self-esteem, especially to unwarranted high self-esteem (that is, narcissism)' (p. 31).[3]

There is no doubt that each of these models provides reasonable explanations of aggression. However, taking on board Anderson and Bushman's (2002) sentiments, perhaps a unifying framework that they call 'the General Aggression Model' (GAM) is needed in order to best understand aggression as a phenomenon.

Anderson and Bushman's general aggression model

The premise of GAM is based on the way knowledge is structured, which according to Anderson and Bushman (2002) is as follows.

- Knowledge is the result of experience.

- Knowledge influences perception at multiple levels, that is, from the very basic to the most complex.

- Knowledge can become automatised as in *doing something without having to think about it.*

- Knowledge is linked to affective, cognitive, and conative domains.

- Knowledge is used to guide people's perception and behaviour to their social as well as physical environment.

In addition to these, Anderson and Bushman (2002) posit that there are three relevant subtypes of knowledge structures and these are 'perceptual schemata',[4] 'personal schemata', and 'behavioural scripts'. Given that schemata or schema is a map or mould for processing information, perceptual schemata would suggest that an individual uses a particular template to view an interaction. For example, a joke could be interpreted as a personal insult. Similarly, personal schema is made up of beliefs that are attributed to people, for example, we may see someone as hostile. Behavioural script is described as 'appropriate sequences of events in a particular context' (Schank & Abelson, 1977, p. 41). The implication is that these can be predetermined and stereotyped sequence of actions that define a well-known situation. According to Anderson and Bushman (2002), behavioural scripts contain information about how people behave under varying circumstances. GAM emphasises the person-situation dynamics through three principal focal points highlighted as INPUTS, ROUTES, and OUTCOMES.

Inputs

Input focuses on person and situation, for example biological, environmental, psychological, and social factors can and do influence aggressive behaviour. These can be clustered under two principal themes of person and situation (see Table 5.6).

Traits

According to Baron and Richardson (1994), informal observation suggests that there are certain characteristics that predispose specific individuals towards or away from aggression. These may relate to some people who are quick tempered by comparison to others who have a high tolerance to frustrations or irritations. It is also well known that certain traits predispose individuals to high levels of aggression. For example, according to Anderson and Bushman (2002), certain types of people who frequently aggress against others do so mainly because of their susceptibility towards hostile attribution, perception, and expectation biases. Moreover, Berkowitz (1993) states that a high proportion of people who abuse the members of their families have persistent inclinations towards violence. According to Loeber and Hay (1997), systematic individual differences in temperament emerge very early in a person's life. For example, in infancy some

Table 5.6 Person- and situation-related factors

Person-related factors	Situation-related factors
Traits	Aggressive cues
Gender	Provocation
Attitudes, values, and beliefs	Frustration
Scripts	Pain and discomfort
	Drugs
	Incentive

babies are less easy to soothe and experience difficulty adapting to the rhythms of social life. Loeber and Hay (1997) suggest that some of the behaviour may be predisposed. This is validated by Emde et al. (1992), who from their longitudinal study reported genetic implication in infants' irritability and expression of negative emotions such as anger.

Gender

It would seem that there are differences in aggressive tendencies between men and women (Anderson & Bushman, 2002). Numerous studies have found that men are more likely to be the aggressors and the victims of direct physical aggression (see Berkowitz, 1993; Campbell, 1995). However, indirect aggression seems to be more common in girls and women than boys and men. Interestingly, various studies have reported that 'women are at least as likely than men to say that they have instigated various aggressive acts, like slapping or throwing things, but that women are more likely to be injured or killed as a result of violence between intimates' (Harris & Knight-Bohnhoff, 1996, p. 28). However, Hennessy and Wiesenthal (2001) support the argument that indirect aggression where other individuals are used to harm a target is more common among females by comparison to males.

Attitudes, values, and beliefs[5]

According to Allport (1935), an attitude is a mental state of readiness that is organised through experience and has a direct influence on an individual's response to all objects to which it is related. Attitudes can be positive and negative. The implication is that people who hold a positive attitude towards aggression and violence are more likely to aggress than those with a negative attitude. Similarly, values are important life goals or societal conditions that are desired by an individual, and these can be both abstract (such as power, control, and domination) and concrete (as in material possessions for example money and land). Therefore, those who seek power, control, and domination are more likely to be aggressive than those who seek peace. Beliefs are subjective ideas and thoughts, the contents of which can be described as true or false. For example, if we believe that aggression pays then it is more likely that we will be prone to aggress. Moreover, one's self-efficaciousness would dictate whether an aggressive act is carried out or not. For example, if we believe that we can successfully execute an aggressive act that will lead to a desired outcome the likelihood is that we will display aggressive behaviour in comparison to others who may not be so confident of their chances of success. According to Huesmann and Guerra (1997), normative belief does predict future level of aggression in that people's own cognition of what is acceptable or unacceptable behaviour tends to dictate what they do. Huesmann and Guerra (1997, p. 409) offer the following predictions:

- People who are more aggressive should have normative beliefs that are more approving of aggression.

- Over time those people with stronger approval-of-aggression normative beliefs should become more aggressive.

- Engaging in aggressive behaviour promotes the development of normative beliefs approving of aggression as a schema.

- An expectation would be that older children and boys believe that aggression is more acceptable.

Scripts

Script as previously explained is a cognitive schema that contains information of how to behave in a particular situation. According to Anderson and Bushman (2002), the scripts that we bring to a social situation influence our readiness for aggression.

Situational factors

Situational factors such as *aggressive cues* are said to prime aggressive thoughts in some individuals. For example, the presence of guns and knives may trigger aggressive thoughts. Exposure to violent films or video games is linked to aggression. Similarly, with *provocation and frustration*[6] come aggressive response. Provocation could be described as the most important single cause of aggression in human. The implication is that people may find it very difficult to restrain themselves when provoked. Personal, clinical observation, and research suggest that *pain and discomfort* can lead to aggressive behaviour (see Berkowitz, 1993b; Anderson et al., 2003). *Drugs* such as alcohol and caffeine are also implicated in aggressive behaviour. However, drugs like these may not be directly responsible for the aggression, but they may reduce the level of tolerance to provocation and frustration. The notion of incentive as a contributory factor for aggression can be see in operant conditioning (discussed earlier in this chapter).

Routes

Anderson and Bushman (2002) contextualise routes as the present internal states. For example, personal and situational factors tend to influence an individual's intrapersonal dynamic cognition (thoughts and beliefs), affect (mood and emotions), and arousal (physiological and psychological). In relation to the notion that exposure to violent films or video games lead to aggressive behaviour, Anderson (1997) states that viewing violent scenes primes related aggressive thoughts in semantic memory[7] through a spreading activation process, thus increasing the probability of aggressive behaviour in response to provocation (whether this is real or imagined) and in turn serves to increase hostile affect.

Outcomes

These according to Anderson and Bushman (2002) vary from automatic to controlled depending on the type of appraisal one engages in. For example, an immediate appraisal of the present internal state will lead to automatic responses where reappraisal makes the response much more controlled.

Functions of anger and aggression

Berkowitz (1993) posits that one of the major questions in the scientific study of aggression is related to its goals. For example, what purpose does aggression serve? 'Do the attackers mainly want to harm their victims, or are they trying to do something else?' (Berkowitz, 1993, p. 7). The implication is that there are specific reasons for the display of aggressive behaviour. Some of these, however, may be outside one's consciousness. Anderson and Bushman (2002) believe that anger plays at least five causal roles in aggression and these are listed below.

1. Anger reduces inhibitions against aggressive retaliation in that it provides a justification for aggressive behaviour. It may also interfere with moral reasoning and rational thinking.

2. Anger allows an individual to maintain an aggressive intention over time. The implication is that individuals come to dwell on their aggressive thought to such an extent that it increases their attention to the provoking events.

3. Anger is used as an information cue in that it informs people about causes, culpability, and possible ways of responding.

4. Anger primes aggressive thoughts, scripts, and associated expressive behaviours.

5. Anger provides the energy for angry behaviour by increasing one's levels of arousal.

The above functions can be clustered under four principal themes and these are ventilation of feeling as in catharsis, defence against anxiety, controlling, and protection.

Management of anger and aggression in self and in others

It could be argued that in order to successfully manage anger in self and in others, one would need to recognise when the expression of anger is maladaptive in the first instance. Individuals will come to realise that interaction with others may be problematic. The starting point of any management programme is with an assessment of the degree to which anger and aggression lead to negative intrapersonal dynamics and interpersonal relationships. There are numerous ways of assessing anger and aggression. Some of these were introduced earlier in this chapter (see Section on 'Anger Profile'). The purpose of profiling one's own anger and stress levels serves to offer valuable information and insight into what may have triggered angry reactions. For example, in assessing *what makes you angry*, your awareness would be raised in relation to the things or events that initiated the anger. There are various inventories or questionnaires that can help to facilitate this process. In fact, Suris et al. (2004) offer an overview of 41 clinical and research instruments that are available to measure anger and aggression. Amongst these are Seigel (1986) and Buss and Perry (1992). Seigel's (1986) multidimensional anger inventory is particularly useful because as she says the inventory is sensitive to the multidimensional nature of the anger construct and addresses the following dimensions: **Frequency** (I get angry more frequently than most people), **Magnitude** (I get so angry, I feel like I might lose control), **Mode of expression** (I am secretly critical of others), **Hostile outlook** (people can bother me just by being around), and **R**ange of anger-eliciting situations (I get angry when I am not given credit for something I have done). Bush and Perry's (1992) Aggression Questionnaire considers four aggression factors and these are **P**hysical (I have become so mad that I have broken things), **V**erbal (I can't help getting into arguments when people disagree with me), **A**nger (I have trouble controlling my temper), and **H**ostility (I wonder why sometimes I feel so bitter about things). Once individuals have established that their anger-aggression dynamics are maladaptive they have two options, they can do nothing or they can attempt to address their issues, bearing in mind that maladaptive behaviour will only serve to escalate the problem.

Managing anger and aggression in self

It could be argued that the starting point of managing anger and aggression in self is to establish the trigger factors. For example, these could be the environment (real or imagined hostility), self (own fears or inadequacies and frustrated needs), and/or others (provocation). Crucial to these are Anderson and Bushman's (2002) notion of perceptual and personal schemata and behavioural scripts. This may mean engaging in the following course of actions.

- Reevaluating and revising one's existing template to view the situation. Put it simply, individuals would need to restructure their thinking and perception. Knowledge structures of anger and aggression should not be allowed to escape conscious awareness. Individuals should constantly reappraise their knowledge structures, thus aiming for more controlled instead of automatic responses. However, the type of controlled responses one would expect is adaptive rather than maladaptive. For example, premeditated retaliation to provocation or harm would be seen as controlled maladaptive response and would be unacceptable. A point to note here is that controlled adaptive response may take time.

- Similarly, individuals would need to reevaluate their scripts with a view to modify or change these.

Managing anger and aggression in others

Managing anger and aggression in others (those accessing health services) would require the same starting point as in establishing the trigger factors (see earlier discussion in relation to some of the possible causes of anger and aggression in health care settings). It could be said that the sudden change in one's health status would be sufficient to explain why one may be angry. From a personal perspective it would not be difficult to imagine the anger I would experience from being a lecturer today and a patient tomorrow. With this in mind, once the trigger factors are identified a degree of self-awareness would need to be employed in managing anger and aggression in others. It can't be emphasised enough that health care practitioners' self-awareness is central to care delivery.

Summary

Anger can be described as one of the most intense of emotions which if not controlled can lead to negative consequences because the underpinning thought is one of attack. Anger does not directly cause aggression but only accompanies the inclination to attack a target. Aggression, on the other hand, is described as a response that delivers an aversive stimulus to another organism. Various forms of aggression are discussed and these range from actively engaging in acts of verbal and/or physical violence to non-involvement as in *doing nothing*. Moreover, numerous theories have been discussed in an attempt to explain the dynamics of anger and aggression. All these theories are valid in their own rights, however, the one that seems to offer a comprehensive explanation is that of Anderson and Bushman's (2002) GAM that emphasises inputs, routes, and outcomes. At least five functions of anger and aggression are highlighted, but these are not always within one's conscious awareness. Managing anger and aggression in self and in others can be said to rest with one's self-awareness.

References

Allport, G. (1935). Attitudes. In C. Murchison (ed.), *Handbook of Social Psychology* (pp. 798–844). Worcester: Clark University Press.

Anderson, C. A. (1997). Effects of violent movies and trait irritability on hostile feelings and aggressive thoughts. *Aggressive Behaviour*, 23, 161–178.

Anderson, C. A. and Bushman, B. J. (2002). Human Aggression. *Annual Review of Psychology*, 53, 27–51.

Anderson, C. A., Berkowitz, L., Donnerstein, E., Heusmann, L. R., Johnson, J. D., Linz, D., Malamuth, N. M., and Wartella, E. (2003). The influence of media violence on youth. *Psychological Science in the Public Interest*, 4(3), 81–110.

Archer, J. (1988). *The Behavioural Biology of Aggression*. Cambridge: Cambridge University Press.

Archer, J. (2006). Testosterone and human aggression: an evaluation of the challenge hypothesis. *Neuroscience and Biobehavioural Reviews*, 30, 319–345.

Aronson, E., Wilson, T. D., and Akert, R. M. (1997). *Social Psychology*. New York: Longman.

Bandura, A. (1973). *Aggression: A Social Learning Analysis*. Englewood Cliffs: Prentice-Hall International, Inc.

Bandura, A. (1986). *Social Foundation of Thought and Action: A Social Cognitive Theory*. Englewood Cliffs: Prentice-Hall.

Bandura, A., Ross, D., and Ross, S. A. (1961). Transmission of aggression through imitation of aggressive models. *Journal of Abnormal and Social Psychology*, 63(3), 575–582.

Bandura, A., Ross, D., and Ross, S. A. (1963). Imitation of film-mediated aggressive models. *Journal of Abnormal and Social Psychology*, 66, 3–11.

Baron, R. A. and Richardson, D. (1994). *Human Aggression*. New York: Plenum.

Berkowitz, L. (1988). Frustrations, appraisals, and aversively stimulated aggression. *Aggressive Behaviour*, 14, 3–11.

Berkowitz, L. (1993a). *Aggression; its Causes, Consequences, and Control*. New York and London: McGraw-Hill.

Berkowitz, L. (1993b). Pain and aggression: some findings and implications. *Motivation and Emotion*, 17, 277–293.

Blum, H. P. (1995). Sanctified aggression, hate, and the alteration of standard and values. In S. Akhter, S. Kramer, and H. Parens (eds.), *The Birth of Hatred: Developmental, Clinical, and Technical Aspects of Intense Aggression* (pp. 15–37). Northvale and London: Jason Aronson Inc.

Bugentall, D. B. and Goodnow, J. J. (1998). Socialisation processes. In W. Damon and N. Eisenberg (eds.), *Handbook of Child Psychology: Social, Emotional, and Personality Development* (Vol. 3, 5th edition, pp. 389–462). New York, Chichester, Weinheim, Brisbane, Singapore, and Toronto: Wiley & Sons, Inc.

Buss, A. H. (1961). *The Psychology of Aggression.* New York: Wiley.

Buss A. H., and Perry, M. P. (1992). The aggression questionnaire. *Journal of Personality and Social Psychology*, 63, 452–459.

Cahagan, J. (1984). *Social Interaction and its Management.* London and New York: Methuen.

Campbell, A. (1995). A few good men: evolutionary psychology and female adolescent aggression. *Ethology and Sociobiology*, 16, 99–123.

Darwin, C. (1859). *On the Origin of the Species.* London: Murray.

Dollard, J., Doob, L. W. Miller, N. E., Mowrer, O. H., and Sears, R. R. (1939). *Frustration and Aggression.* New Haven: Yale University Press.

Dubin, W. R. (1989). The role of fantasies countertransference and psychological defenses in patient violence. *Hospital and Community Psychiatry*, 40, 1280–1283.

Dutton, D. G. (1999). Traumatic origins of intimate rage. *Aggression and Violent Behaviour*, 4(4), 431–447.

Dutton, D. G., Van Ginkle, C., and Starzomski A. (1995). The role of shame and guilt in the intergenerational transmission of abusiveness. *Violence and Victims*, 10, 121–131.

Emde, R. N., Plomin, R., Robinson, J., Corley, R., DeFries, J., et al. (1992). Temperament, emotion, and cognition at fourteen months: the MacArthur Longitudinal Twin Study. *Child Development*, 63, 1437–1455.

Farrell, G. A. (1999). Aggression in clinical settings: nurses' views- a follow-up study. *Journal of Advanced Nursing*, 29(3), 532–541.

Farrell, G. A. (2001). From tall poppies to squashed weeds: why don't nurses pull together more? *Journal of Advanced Nursing*, 35(1), 26–33.

Freud, S. (1915). Instincts and their vicissitudes. In *The Standard Edition of the Complete Psychological Works of Sigmund Freud* (pp. 110–140). Translated from German under the general editorship of James Strachey in collaboration with Anna Freud assisted by Alix Strachey and Alan Tyson. Volume XIV (1914–1916) *On the History of the Psycho-Analytic Movement. Papers on Metapsychology and Other Works.*

Freud, S. (1920). *Beyond the Pleasure Principle.* New York: Bantam Books.

Freud, S. (1930). *Civilization and its Discontents.* London: Hogarth Press.

Freud, S. (1993). *Historical and Expository Works on Psychoanalysis* (Vol. 15). The Penguin Freud Library. Translated from German under the general editorship of James Strachey. This volume edited by Albert Dickson. London: Penguin Books.

Geen, R. G. (2001). *Human Aggression.* Buckingham and Philadelphia: Open University Press.

Gershoff, E. T. (2002). Corporal punishment by parents and associated child behaviours and experiences: a meta-analytical and theoretical review. *Psychological Bulletin*, 128(4), 539–579.

Gillig, P. M., Markert, R., Barron, J., and Coleman, F. (1998). A comparison of staff and patient perceptions of the causes and cures of physical aggression on a psychiatric unit. *Psychiatric Quarterly*, 69(1), 45–60.

Goffman, I. (1967). *Interaction Ritual.* New York: Anchor.

Gustafson, R. (1986). Human physical aggression as a function of frustration: role of aggressive cues. *Psychological Reports*, 59, 103–110.

Harris, M. B. and Knight-Bohnhoff, K. (1996). Gender and aggression II: personal aggressiveness. *Sex Roles*, 35(1/2), 27–42.

Health Services Advisory Committee (1987). *Violence to Staff in Health Services. Health and Safety Commission.* London: HMSO.

Hennessy, D. A. and Wiesenthal, D. L. (2001). Gender, driver, aggression, and driver violence: an applied evaluation. *Sex Roles*, 44(11/12), 661–676.

Hoffman, M. L. (1960). Power assertion by the parent and its impact on the child. *Child Development*, 31, 129–143.

Howe, M. J. A. (1980). *The Psychology of Human Learning*. New York: Harper and Row.

Huesmann, L. R. and Guerra, N. G. (1997). Children's normative beliefs about aggression and aggressive behaviour. *Journal of Personality and Social Psychology*, 72, 408–419.

Huesmann, L. R., Eron. L. D., and Dubow, E. (2002). Childhood predictors of adult criminality: are all risk factors reflected in childhood aggressiveness? *Criminal Behaviour and Mental Health*, 12, 185–208.

Kernberg, O. F. (1995). Hatred as a core affect of aggression. In S. Akhter, S. Kramer, and H. Parens (eds.), *The Birth of Hatred: Developmental, Clinical, and Technical Aspects of Intense Aggression* (pp. 53–82). Northvale and London: Jason Aronson Inc.

Krahé, B. (2001). *The social Psychology of Aggression*. Hove: Psychology Press Ltd.

Kurlowitz, L. H. (1990). Violence in the emergency department. *American Journal of Nursing*, 90, 34–39.

Lazar, R. (2003). Knowing hatred. *International Journal of Psychoanalysis*, 84, 405–425.

Loeber, R. and Hay, D. (1997). Key issues in the development of aggression and violence from childhood to early adulthood. *Annual Review of Psychology*, 48, 371–410.

Lorenz, K. (1966). *On Aggression*. London: Methuen.

Miller, N. E. (1941). The Frustration-Aggression Hypothesis. *Psychological Review*, 48, 337–342.

Naish, J., Carter, Y. H., Gray, R. W., Stevens, T., Tissier, J. M., and Gantley, M. M. (2002). Brief encounters of aggression and violence in primary care: a team approach to coping strategies. *Family Practice*, 19, 504–510.

Newsom, C., Flavell, J. E., and Rincover, A. (1983). The side effects of punishment. In S. Axelrod and J. Apsche (eds.), *The Effect of Punishment on Human Behaviour* (pp. 285–316). New York: Academic Press.

Pavlov, I. P. (1927). *Conditioned Reflexes*. New York: Oxford University Press.

Renfrew, J. W. (1997). *Aggression and its Causes: A Biopsychosocial Approach*. New York: Oxford University Press.

Rippon, T. J. (2000). Aggression and violence in health care professions. *Journal of Advanced Nursing*, 31 (2), 452–460.

Rungapadiachy, D. M. (2003). *The Role of the Mental Health Nurse: a Comparison of the Perceptions of Mental Health Nurses at Three Levels of Experience (Pre-Post Registration, and Experienced Mental Health Nurses)*. Unpublished PhD Thesis. University of Leeds, Leeds.

Schank, R. and Abelson, R. (1977). *Scripts, Plans, Goals, and Understanding: An Inquiry into Human Knowledge Structures*. Hillsdale: Lawrence Erlbaum Associates Publishers.

Secker, J., Benson, A., Balfe, E., Lipsedge, M., Robinson, S., and Walker, J. (2004). Understanding the social context of violent and aggressive incidents on an inpatient unit. *Journal of Psychiatric and Mental Health Nursing*, 11, 172–178.

Seigel, J. M. (1986). The multidimensional anger inventory. *Journal of Personality and Social Psychology*, 51(1), 191–200.

Skinner, F. B. (1953). *Science and Human Behaviour*. New York: Macmillan.

Skinner, B. F. (1971). *Beyond Freedom and Dignity*. New York: Knopf.

Suris, A., Lind, L., Emmett, G., Borman, P. D., Kashner, M., and Barratt, E. S. (2004). Measures of aggressive behaviour: overview of clinical and research instruments. *Aggression and Violent Behaviour*, 9, 165–227.

Thorndike, E. (1932). *The Fundamentals of Learning*. New York: Teachers College Press.

Todorov, A. and Bargh, J. A. (2002). Automatic sources of aggression. *Aggression and Violent Behaviour*, 7, 53–68.

Whittington, R. W., Shuttleworth, S., and Hill, L. (1996). Violence to staff in a general hospital setting. *Journal of Advanced Nursing*, 24, 326–333.

Wiener, J. (1998). Under the volcano: varieties of anger and their transformation. *Journal of Analytical Psychology*, 43, 493–508.

Wingfield, J. C., Hegner, R. E., Duffy, A. M., and Ball, G. F. (1990). The 'challenge hypothesis': theoretical implications for patterns of testosterone secretion, mating systems, and breeding strategies. *The American Naturalist*, 136, 829–846.

Winstanley, S. and Whittington, R. (2004). Aggression towards health care staff in a UK general hospital: variation among professions and departments. *Journal of Clinical Nursing*, 13, 3–10.

Yanay, N. (2002). Hatred as ambivalence. *Theory, Culture & Society*, 19(3), 71–88.

PART

III

Communication, Engagement, and the Helping Relationship

Involving patients in their care is regarded as a means of enhancing the quality of services offered to them. Evidence suggests that participation encourages patients' self-worth and empowerment, thus leading to a greater sense of control. Moreover, some have argued that people have a greater sense of efficacy when they come to believe that self-involvement makes a difference in how they are cared for. It becomes clear therefore that engagement can only be a positive move towards health care delivery. Recognising the need to collaborate with patients, the NHS Plan (2000) set out by the British Government proposes that 'patients will have far greater information about how they can look after their own health and about their local health services. The "Expert Patient" Programme will be extended. The National Institute for Clinical Excellence will publish patient friendly versions of all its clinical guidelines. Patients will be helped to navigate the maze of health information through the development of NHS Direct online' (Department of Health, 2000, p. 91). The very essence of engagement would seem to rest with actively involving patients in every aspect of their care through easy access to information. However, according to Thomson, Bowling, and Moss (2001), truly involving patients in treatment decisions will require fundamental review and reappraisal of some of the stated objectives of health care. The implication is that giving information may not be sufficient to translate the notion of engagement in decision making into reality. The treatment of hypertension is considered as a case in point. Thomson, Bowling, and Moss (2001) argue that the commonly stated objective of treating hypertension in a population of patients is to reduce the morbidity and mortality from illnesses such as stroke and coronary heart disease. This would mean identifying people who are at risk and treating any one whose blood pressure is considered to be 'high'. The implication here is that those people who were 'symptom free' before will now be clustered under the 'hypertensive' brackets and deemed 'ill' and treatment prescribed. Thomson, Bowling, and Moss (2001, p. i1) ask the following questions. 'But what if patients themselves were to decide on their own treatment after receiving full information on the risks and benefits? Would they make the same decisions as their doctors would advise?' According to Finlay et al. (2000), this may not be the case, as it would appear that patients were less likely to want antihypertensive therapy, especially when baseline cardiovascular risks were low. Proposing a new method of working is one thing and implementing it is a totally different thing altogether. The complexity of the notion of engagement therefore should not be underestimated. The ensuing chapters attempt to address some of the issues relating to engagement, such as language (Chapter 6), intrapersonal communication (Chapter 7), interpersonal communication and skills (Chapter 8), and engagement and developing relationship (Chapter 9).

References

Department of Health (2000). *NHS Plan 2000: A Plan for Investment, a Plan for Reform.* Norwich: HMSO.

Finlay, A. M., O'Connor, A. M., Wells, G., Grover, S. A., and Laupacis, A. (2000). When should hypertension be treated? The different perspectives of Canadian family physicians and patients. *Canadian Medical Association Journal*, 163(4), 403–408.

Thomson, R., Bowling, A. and Moss, F. (2001). Engaging patients in decisions: a challenge to health care delivery and public health. *Quality in Health care*, 10 (Supplement 1), i1.

The Use of Language and Self-Awareness

Jack Morris and Dev M. Rungapadiachy

OBJECTIVES

After reading this chapter you should be able to

- Discuss the formation of language from a bio-psycho-social perspective.

- Demonstrate an understanding of how language conveys meaning.

- Reflect upon ways language is expressed within health care practice.

Introduction

Described as the faculty of making signs, language can be seen as a forerunner to the notion of human communication. The word language has its origin in French *langue* and Latin *lingua*, both terms taken to mean tongue, and is described as a system made up of words, signs, sounds, and gestures for conveying meaning and understanding to one another. Language is primarily a tool for communicating thought, for example, when individuals say *I can't find the words*, what they are really saying is *I can't think*. According to Romanes (1984), the faculty of language is the faculty of making signs that occurs when a person becomes self-conscious. Romanes (1984) distinguishes four stages of sign making and these are inductive (long before a child is able to speak, he or she makes significant tones and gestures, for example, pointing to an object of desire), denotative (names that have been learnt by association are used as expression but thoughts are not implicated), connotative (this consists of an extension of the meaning of that name to other things of similar resemblance), and denominative (names are given to objects consciously and are dependent on the attainment of self-consciousness). The first three of these stages are said to be common to both human beings and animals but advance much further in the growing child than they do in any animal. The fourth stage, denominative, is distinctly a human attribute, thus inextricably linked with society. Moreover, language and other social activity are mutually related (Cherry, 1966). The implication is that 'the interests and needs of the day force changes upon the language and, in turn, the language is dominant over our thought' (Cherry, 1966, p. 32). Attempts are made within this chapter to explore the concept of language and issues related to its use in health care settings.

The formation of language

Language has two components and these are production and comprehension. The production aspect of language starts with a thought, which is then translated into a word (phrase or sentence). This word is then expressed in sound. Comprehension on the other hand starts with the hearing of the sound, where meaning is attached in the form of word in order to create a phrase or sentence. A spoken language therefore could be considered as a system of sounds, the basic unit of which is called phoneme. Phoneme therefore can be seen as meaningless sound for example C, M, and S. The smallest unit of a meaningful sound is called morpheme, for example CAT, MAT, and SAT. The structure of a word is governed by morphological rules for example by adding an 's' to some morphemes their meanings could be translated from singular to plural as in CATS and MATS. When words are grouped together the sentiment that they convey can range from meaningless to meaningful depending on their order of arrangements. For example, take a look at the words THE, MAT, CAT, THE, ON, SAT. Grouped in the order as they appear (that is, THE MAT CAT THE ON SAT), they would be described as meaningless. However, when arranged in a different sequence, for example, THE CAT SAT ON THE MAT, the overall meaning is very clear. This type of arrangement of words that convey meaning is referred to as syntax.

The development of language

The origin of language is variously suggested to emerge in order to provide information about the spatial aspects of the environment (O'Keefe & Nadel, 1978) or to maintain the social fabric of increasingly large groups of hominoids, for example, replacing grooming activities and providing a way of spreading gossip (Dunbar, 1996). There does not appear to be a consensus of opinion as to when human species constructed (rudimentary) language sounds and corresponding gestures. One suggestion is, evolutionary speaking, language is a relatively recent phenomenon, unique to human species that emerged some 100–150,000 years ago as a by-product of the brain reaching a certain critical level of complexity (Chomsky, 1975). Stein (2003) summarises three possible suggestions as to why linguistic communication could have been important for our distant ancestors.

1. Linguistic communication enabled the shared use of tools. Language was thus used to explain their employment in hunting or self-preservation.

2. Language evolved as a method of planning the best strategy for hunting prey. Within this process there could be the development of abstract thought such as predictions and strategies for hunting.

3. Language development was a requirement to find a mate.

Moreover, these adaptations took place over millions of years. Whatever ideas, speculations, or facts can be gleaned from an appreciation of language development in ancient times, we may still possess those earlier forms of communication. Given that anecdotal information is limited, there is no way of knowing how our ancestors expressed emotions such as pain, distress, happiness, and sexual attraction. If tribal behaviour is anything to go by, survival (attacks from others), procreation (attraction to others), and continued existence (food, warmth, and shelter), then ways of communicating understanding through grunts, groans, and gestures could have become a valuable way of signalling a variety of intentions to other members. Gesture as a form of language is the most likely predecessor to spoken language (Corballis, 1999). From what is known, language evolves from a complex and dynamic series of biological, psychological, and social activities, resulting in varying ways of demonstrating understanding, meaning, and expressing feelings to others. Very few would contradict the importance of biology to language development.

Biological basis of language

Perhaps one of the easiest ways of discussing the biological basis of language is to consider the localisation of function in the brain, which as is well documented is divided into two sections, commonly known as hemispheres and these are symmetrical (see Figure 6.1).

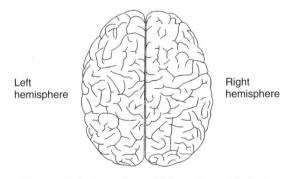

Left
hemisphere

Right
hemisphere

Figure 6.1 The right and left hemisphere of the brain.

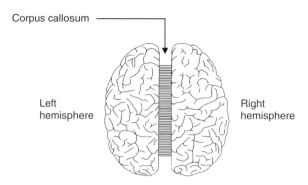

Figure 6.2 The corpus callosum connects the right and left hemispheres together.

These two hemispheres are connected to each other by a thick band of fibres called corpus callosum (see Figure 6.2). This pathway is responsible for the intercommunication that takes place between these hemispheres. Each hemisphere is responsible for different and specialised functions, for example, the left hemisphere is responsible for number skills, reasoning ability, and right-handed control.

Similarly, the left hemisphere is responsible for insight, awareness of art, power of imagination, music awareness, and left-hand control. According to Harley (2001), for the majority (96%) of right-handed people language functions are predominantly situated in the left hemisphere. However, a contemporary review on how language is organised concludes that the right hemisphere also makes a substantial contribution to many aspects of language comprehension and this is seen as critical to social communication (Bookheimer, 2002). Knowledge of these neurological processes have been enhanced with the advent of brain imaging techniques, allowing an understanding of the relationships between specific areas of the brain and the language functions they serve. The advancements in brain imaging, for example positron emission tomography (PET),[1] employs a scanner to detect injected radioactive materials and provide an image of brain activity. Whereas, functional magnetic resonance imaging (fMRI)[2] uses radio frequency signals produced by displaced radio waves in the magnetic field to detect changes in blood flow providing an anatomical and functional view of the brain. A significant problem when investigating brain imaging is that these results can often be difficult to interpret. The main approach used is called *subtraction* where images from one task, for example reading silently, is subtracted from a second image, reading loudly, in order to identify where the critical difference between the two is located.

Over 150 years of research into the organisation of language within the brain is based upon a lesion deficit approach, which infers the functional significance of an area through observation of deficit following either temporary or permanent brain lesions. Language deficit or impairment due to brain damage caused by a lesion, head injury, or burst blood vessels is known as aphasia. There are two types of aphasia: expressive and receptive. Each relates to the location of the damage. Paul Broca (1861), a French neurologist, having observed several of his patients with

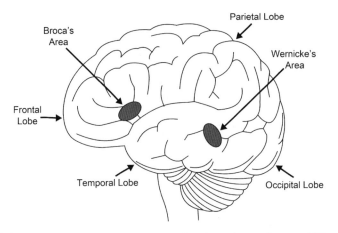

Figure 6.3 Lateral view of the left hemisphere of the brain showing Broca and Wernicke's area.

damage to a specific area (came to be known as Broca's area) in the left temporal lobe of the brain (see Figure 6.3) concluded that these patients were suffering from expressive aphasia (inability to speak). However, their ability to understand remained intact. This condition became known as Broca's aphasia. A contemporary view has argued that Broca's area can be subdivided into three regions, each serving a specific function (Bookheimer, 2002). These are as follows.

1. One area can be found in the posterior and superior part and said to be implicated in sound structure (phonology).

2. The second area is located within the anterior and ventral part and is concerned with the meaning of words (referred to as semantic).

3. The third sits between the first two regions and is involved in the meaning conveyed by sentence structure (syntax).

Wernicke (1874), a German neurologist, discovered another area in left hemisphere of the brain but further down from Broca's area into the temporal lobe (Wernicke's area see Figure 6.3) where damage resulted in receptive aphasia. This means that people with this condition would not be able to understand the meaning of words. They would, however, have no difficulty articulating words although these can be meaningless. Receptive aphasia became known as Wernicke's aphasia.

The Wernicke–Geschwind model

Wernicke–Geschwind's model (Geschwind, 1979) was the first model to explain the organisation of language in the brain. The production and comprehension of language are arranged in the following way. When someone speaks, we receive this information from our ears and it travels through to the primary auditory area (see Figure 6.4).

However, in order to comprehend what we have heard, speech content needs to be transmitted to Wernicke's area (which is responsible for language

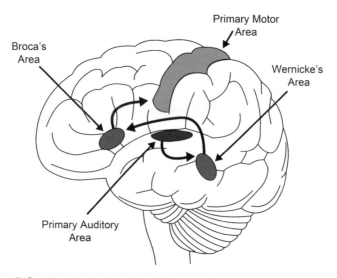

Figure 6.4 Wernicke–Geschwind model showing the pathways for language production and comprehension on hearing a speech.

comprehension) where word meanings are extracted. Moreover, if we want to speak, for example, in response to what we have heard, then information from Wernicke's area would need to be sent to the Broca's area (responsible for language expression). Broca's area in turn sends information to the motor area (Figure 6.4) in order to drive the physiological mechanisms for speech sound. For example, the lips, tongue, and larynx are activated to speak.

A similar dynamic is at play for speaking a written word. However, in this instance information is captured visually by our eyes and registered in the primary visual area (Figure 6.5). This information is relayed to the angular

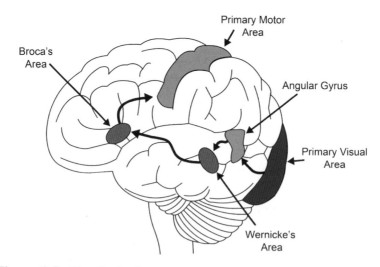

Figure 6.5 Wernicke–Geschwind model showing the pathways for language production and comprehension on seeing a written word.

gyrus where the arrangements of letters and their shapes (that is, visual coding for words) are compared with how they sound (that is, acoustic coding). As soon as a match is found, this information is transmitted to Wernicke's area where meaning is subtracted. From here on the same process is involved as with hearing a spoken word. That is, word meanings are transmitted to Broca's area and in turn to primary motor area and hence the formation of speech sounds.

Critical period in language development

Critical period can be described as a stage in development where an organism is at its optimum to learn a new behaviour. The implication is that if language has not developed by the time this critical period has expired then its development becomes problematic. According to Lenneberg (1967), the development of language is contingent upon a certain level of maturation and growth. For example, between

> the ages of two and three years language emerges by an interaction of maturation and self-programmed. Between the ages of three and the early teens the possibility for primary language acquisition continues to be good; the individual appears to be most sensitive to stimuli at this time and to preserve some innate flexibility for the organization of brain functions to carry out the complex integration of subprocesses necessary for the smooth elaboration of speech and language.
>
> (Lenneberg, 1967, p. 158)

Moreover, it would appear that the ability to respond to the physiological demands of verbal behaviour declines after puberty. The implication according to Lenneberg is that if language skills are not acquired by then, production of language is usually lost forever. Lenneberg (1967) does acknowledge that the picture is much more complicated than stated as the 'maturational data for the end of the critical period is more difficult to interpret' (p. 168). The case of Genie goes some way to support Lenneberg's critical hypothesis theory. According to Curtiss (1977), Genie suffered extreme abuse, neglect, and isolation possibly from birth through to 13½ years old by her father. 'In the house Genie was confined to a small bedroom, harnessed to an infant's potty seat. Genie's father sewed the harness, himself; unclad except for the harness, Genie was left to sit on that chair. Unable to move anything except her fingers and hands, feet and toes, Genie was left to sit, tied-up, hour after hour, often into the night, day after day, month after month, year after year' (Curtiss, 1977, p. 5). Moreover, at night when Genie was not forgotten in her potty seat, she was transferred to a straight jacket. She had no auditory stimulation. It would appear that the only contact Genie had with others was when her mother fed her and 'occasionally when her father and older brother barked at her like dogs' (Harley, 2001, p. 69). As a result of this Genie's language was abnormal. 'Her language resembles that of other cases of right-hemisphere language as well as the language of those generally acquiring language outside of the "critical period" '(Curtiss, 1977, p. 234).

If this is the case, one may well ask, *how does one explain the acquisition of a second language?* According to Hakuta, Bialystok, and Wiley (2003), there is sufficient empirical evidence to claim that there is an age-related decline in the success with which individuals master a second language (see Flege, Yeni-Komshian, & Liu, 1999; Steven, 1999). Johnson and Newport (1989) propose two versions to explain the critical period hypothesis, the exercise hypothesis and the maturational state hypothesis.

1. The exercise hypothesis states that early in life people have a superior capacity for acquiring languages. However, this capacity will only remain intact throughout life provided it is utilised during that time. One can deduce from this that children will be superior to adults in acquiring a first language. If individuals are not exposed to a first language during their childhood the likelihood is that they will not be proficient at any language in future. Acquiring a first language during childhood means one's capacity to acquire language will remain intact throughout life, thus learning a second language should not be problematic for either children or adults. The exercise hypothesis would equate to the notion of *use it or lose it.*

2. The maturational state hypothesis proposes that early in life people have a superior capacity for acquiring languages. This capacity disappears or declines with maturation. The implication is that there is no guarantee that if individuals have acquired a first language early in life they will have the capacity to learn a second language later in life. It would seem that the maturational state hypothesis favours children at learning both a first and second language better than adults. The maturational hypothesis would equate to the notion of *too late to teach old dog new tricks.*

Psychological basis of language

It is argued that the psychological basis of language rests principally within cognitive development. According to Kolb and Whishaw (2003) the first person, who identified stages in cognitive development was Jean Piaget. In fact, Piaget states that there are four stages of cognitive development and these are sensori-motor, preoperational, concrete operational, and formal operational (see Table 6.1 for an overview of their defining characteristics).

Piaget (1952) argues that the origin of thoughts and intellectual processes is firmly imbedded in what he called schema (schemata in plural). Schema is described as hypothetical cognitive structures that people use to perceive, organise, process, and use information about the world (Hjelle & Ziegler, 1992). Inhelder (1969) sees schema as merely a simplified imagined representation of the result of a specific action. The implication is that self-expression and communication are dictated by individuals' cognitive structures of their language. For example, we will label things the only way we know how unless of course we are taught differently. Schema, therefore, could be seen as the foundation for thoughts. According to Piaget, three processes are important for cognitive development and these are assimilation, accommodation, and equilibration (Siegler, 1991). Described as *the taking on of new information*, assimilation helps individuals transform this information so that they fit within their existing schema.

Table 6.1 An overview of the defining characteristics of the four stages in cognitive development

	Stages and typical age	Defining characteristics
1	Sensori-motor (birth to 2 years)	Behaviour is organised around sensory and motor processes. Action starts from being accidental to purposeful, hence the child recognises self as an agent of action. Relationships between actions and outcomes are established as in cause and effect. 'Sudden comprehension' or insight is developed (see Kohler, 1925). Concept of object permanence is grasped, for example, the child recognises that an object still exists even though it is out of sight
2	Preoperational (2 years to 6 or 7 years)	Acquisition of representational skills through symbols, mental imagery, and drawing. The most dramatic growth is said to take place in the area of language (Siegler, 1991). However, thinking is egocentric (as in self-centred). The implication is that children of these ages are only able to see things from their own viewpoint. Moreover, they lack the ability to grasp the concept of conservation. This means that they can't recognise that the physical properties of things (amount, size, volume, and weight) remain the same even though their shapes or appearances may change
3	Concrete operational (6 or 7 to 11 or 12 years)	The notion of conservation is grasped. Children become less egocentric. They are able to solve problems that involve concrete objects but are not able to deal in abstract. They can focus on more than one dimension of a problem
4	Formal operational (11 or 12 years through to adulthood and old age) (Siegler, 1991)	This stage marks the start of abstract thinking and children are able to deal in abstract as well as solve problems mentally. Thought becomes the instrument for logic and reasoning. For example, they can work with hypothetical concepts, deductive reasoning, make inferences to arrive at conclusions, and generate and test hypotheses

Accommodation, according to Hunt (1969), can be defined as the modification made to an existing schema 'or in a conceptual operation or construction, that comes about in the course of encounters with new circumstances where the existing organization does not quite fit' (Elkind & Flavell, 1969, p. 9). There seems to be a clear interplay between both these terms in that accommodation can't take place without assimilation. However, assimilation can only be recognised as having taken place when, as Hunt (1969) states, an accommodative change in behaviour or thought as reflected in language generalises to a new situation. The notion of equilibration is similar to adaptation in that it involves both assimilation and accommodation. According to Siegler (1991), Piaget considered development to be the formation of more stable equilibriums between children's cognitive system and the external world. The implication is that children's perception of the world would be much more in keeping with reality. Equilibration is said to occur in three phases. 'First, children are satisfied with their mode of thought and therefore are in a state of equilibrium. Then they become aware of shortcomings in their existing thinking and are dissatisfied. This constitutes a state of disequilibrium. Finally, they adopt a more sophisticated mode of thought that eliminates the shortcomings of the old one'

(Siegler, 1991, p. 23). For example, Bart sees a big white horse and calls it a *horse*. When he sees a small black horse, Bart still calls it a *horse*. This would suggest that Bart has assimilated the concept of *horse*. Now, if when he sees a donkey Bart says 'horse', we would rightly assume that he has no schema of donkey. Marje would then say to Bart, *No Bart, that's not a horse, that's a donkey.* With the horse, Bart was in a state of equilibrium, the donkey, however, pushes him into disequilibrium because he is faced with what he sees as contradictory information. When Marje points out the defining characteristics between a horse and a donkey and Bart is able to differentiate between the two animals, he would regain his state of equilibrium. It could be argued that both assimilation and accommodation are key concepts in changing individuals' attitude towards how illness is perceived and labels ascribed to people. The transition from witch to service user would have meant that society has had to reorganise its schema to fit the information or as Kring et al. (2007) state 'construes the information in such a way as to fit the schema' (p. 48). Contemporary thinking and the language we use in relation to mental illness have thus seen a radical change. It is interesting to note, however, how the inclusion or exclusion of one or two words can significantly influence an individual's intra-interpersonal dynamics,[3] thus impacting on health care delivery as examplified in Exercise 1.

EXERCISE 1

This activity is structured in three stages. However, you would need to address each stage separately.

In your professional capacity, you are asked to care for:

  1. A 25-year-old female prostitute who is HIV positive.

Describe your feelings, thoughts, and actions. Then move to stage 2 and still in your professional capacity, you are asked to care for

  2. A 25-year-old female microbiologist who is HIV positive.

Again describe your thoughts, feeling, and actions.

  3. A 25-year-old female doctor who is HIV positive as a result of a sexual assault.

And the same for stage 3.

We could go on omitting word or replacing one for another and one argument is that as we add or remove these descriptive words our thoughts, feelings, and possibly our action will change depending on our ability to assimilate and accommodate information that forces us to view people the way we do. A typical response to stage one of Exercise 1 could be, *well, if you play with fire then expect to get burnt.* The response to stage two might be something like, *the nature of the job meant that she should have been more careful.* In stage three we are most likely to feel, *what an awful thing to happen to a young woman.* The terms *prostitute, microbiologist, doctor,* and *sexual assault* influence our responses.

Egocentric and socialised language

According to Piaget (1932), the functions of children's language can be clustered into two principal themes and these are egocentric and socialised language. Egocentric language emerges during the preoperational stage. The notion of egocentric thinking as described earlier (see Table 6.1) suggests that an individual is not able to appreciate other people points of view. Here, the child 'does not bother to know to whom he is speaking nor whether he is being listened to. He talks either for himself or for the pleasure of associating anyone who happens to be there with the activity of the moment' (Piaget, 1932, p. 9). Egocentric characteristics can be seen in the following behaviour.

- The child only speaks about himself or herself.

- No attempt is made to place himself or herself at the point of view of the listener.

- The listener only serves as an audience and at that 'the child asks for no more than an apparent interest, though he has the illusion (except perhaps in pure soliloquy if even then) of being heard and understood. He feels no desire to influence his hearer nor to tell him anything; not unlike a certain type of drawing-room conversation where every one talks about himself and no one listens' (Piaget, 1932, p. 9).

Exercise 2 encourages awareness of language used by self and others.

EXERCISE 2

Piaget's quote in the last bullet point above clearly shows that egocentric language is not confined solely to children in the preoperational stage. Identify at least one interaction where:

1. You engaged in egocentric language.

2. Your colleagues, friends, partners, or mum, dad, or anyone else who have engaged in egocentric language.

Piaget (1932) lists egocentric speech into three categories: repetition, monologue, and dual or collective monologues.

1. Repetition is in the form of echolalia, for example the child may repeat words or syllables for the sake of pleasure of talking and not necessarily directing at others.

2. In monologue it is as if the child is thinking aloud.

3. In dual or collective monologues (in pairs or groups) the point of view of the other person is not taken into account. Their presence only serves as a stimulus.

Socialised language, as the term suggests, involves reciprocity between two or more individuals whereby thoughts and feelings are exchanged during an interaction. The child, as Piaget (1932, pp. 9–10) states, 'exchanges his thoughts with others, either by telling his hearer something that will interest him and influence his actions, or by an actual interchange of ideas by argument or even by collaboration in pursuit of a common aim'. The defining characteristics of socialised language are in the form of

1. Adapted information (the point of view of other is taken into consideration during the exchanges).

2. Criticism (these may take the form of giving information to suggest one's superiority at the expense of others. It could be argued that this is not an uncommon practice among adults).

3. Commands, requests, and threats between parties concerned.

4. Questioning one another.

5. Answers to real questions.

One of the principal themes in the psychological contribution to the development of language is that thought shapes language. Some would argue that language development occurs in the context of meaningful social interaction (Harley, 2001). Others would say that people with different linguistic and cultural backgrounds think differently (Carroll, 1999). An example is offered by Haffner (1992), who states that 'Latinos feel they should agree with physicians out of politeness and respect, even when they really disagree or do not understand the issues involved. They expect physicians to make the decisions for them and do not understand why they are asked to make choices' (p. 257). Haffner (1992) concludes that language and cultural issues are intermixed. There is no doubt that socialised language develops through interaction with others. The implication is that biological and psychological explanations of language development may not be sufficient to fully grasp the phenomenon of language without exploring its social basis.

Social basis of language

According to Sapir (1929), it would be an illusion to believe that people adjust to the demand of the world (reality) without the use of language. Moreover, linguistic symbolism is a prerequisite to defining the essence of a culture. Language is not merely an accidental means of solving specifics problems of communication nor is it inherent as, for example, in being able to walk.

To put it concisely, walking is an inherent, biological function of man. Eliminate society and there is every reason to believe that he will learn to walk, if indeed, he survives at all. But it is just as certain that he will never learn to talk, that is communicate ideas according the traditional system of a particular society.

(Sapir, 1970, pp. 3–4)

Sapir (1970) believes that language has a setting and the people who speak it belong to a race with their unique physical characteristics that set them apart from other races. Language is thus seen as a non-instinctive method of communication that is produced by symbols but not necessarily implicating thought. However, to think without language may be seen as an illusion because 'no sooner do we try to put an image into conscious relation with another than we find ourselves slipping into a silent flow of words' (Sapir, 1921, p. 15). The dynamic between thought and language was extended by Benjamin Whorf (1956), one of Sapir's students, in his well-known theory of linguistic relativity, the Sapir–Whorf hypothesis.

Sapir–Whorf hypothesis

This explanation is based on our interpretation of Sapir–Whorf hypothesis and bearing in mind as Kay and Kempton (1984) state, 'their writings are notorious for being subject to multiple interpretations' (p. 75). The principal sentiment of Sapir–Whorf hypothesis is that language shapes thought. More importantly, the language a culture uses determines the way its members interpret information about the world. Moreover, differences among languages spoken in different cultures lead to corresponding differences in the way its members perceive the world (Siegler, 1991). The implication is that language does not only relate to thinking but it also determines people's perception of their reality. For example, Whorf states,

> we dissect nature along lines laid down by our native languages. The categories and types that we isolate from the world of phenomena we do not find there because they stare every observer in the face; on the contrary, the world is presented in a kaleidoscope flux of impressions which has to be organized by our minds – and this means largely by the linguistic systems in our minds. We cut nature up, organize it into concepts, and ascribe significances as we do, largely because we are parties to an agreement to organize it in this way – an agreement that holds throughout our speech community and is codified in the patterns of our language. The agreement is, of course, an implicit and unread one, BUT ITS TERMS ARE ABSOLUTELY OBLIGATORY; we cannot talk at all except by subscribing to the organization and classification of data which the agreement decrees.
>
> (Whorf, 1956, pp. 213–214).

This is an interesting concept, as it would appear that our perception is moulded by the society we ascribe to which, in turn, is shaped by its very own linguistic system. It is not our intention here to critique Sapir–Whorf hypothesis as numerous attempts have already been made. Moreover, according to Brown (1976), it has all been said by Lenneberg (1953). Assuming that Sapir–Whorf hypothesis is true and that the structure of an individual's native language significantly influences, if not fully determines his or her view of the world, what then are implications for health care delivery? Consider Exercise 3.

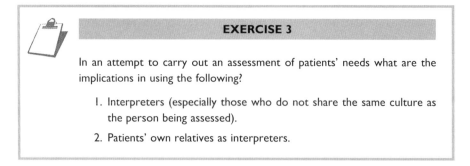

In an attempt to carry out an assessment of patients' needs what are the implications in using the following?

1. Interpreters (especially those who do not share the same culture as the person being assessed).

2. Patients' own relatives as interpreters.

No doubt there are numerous implications in using interpreters, and in fact it could be said that professional interpreters contribute greatly to enhancing the quality of care delivery by virtue of their ability to add to an accurate assessment of health care needs. However, there are instances where the use of professional interpreters has been detrimental to patient care because the latter were unfamiliar with medical terminologies. One such example reported in Porter-O'Grady (2003) highlights an incident where the translator instructed a mother to put the oral antibiotic amoxicillin into her child's ears to treat an ear infection. Here, it may not be difficult to imagine how this error could have happened when we consider the words *ORAL* and *AURAL*. Both words have similar pronunciations. However, oral pertains to the mouth whereas aural relates to the ear. It may well be that the interpreter could have interpreted oral to mean aural. A simple mistake of words one may say. However, the outcome could have been serious. It could be argued that using patient's relative as interpreter is both convenient and economical to health care trusts. However, its value to either patients or their relatives is questionable. See for example Haffner (1992)[4] who gave two accounts that clearly demonstrate the detrimental effect of using patient's relative as interpreters. Haffner (1992) describes a 50-year-old Mexican woman who invented other symptoms to justify her visits to the doctor because she was too embarrassed to disclose to her 35-year-old son (who was also acting as the interpreter) that she has a fistula in her rectum. The second account concerns a 7-year-old girl who was used as an interpreter for her mum during an ultrasound examination and was told by the doctor to tell her mum 'that the baby (her little brother to be) is dead' (Haffner, 1992, p.257). These may have been extreme cases; however, they do illustrate that interpretation is much more than a question of translation. Language and health care are discussed later in this chapter.

The acquisition of language

According to Chomsky (1965, p. 30), the prerequisite to learning language rests with the child's ability to posses the following skills.

- A technique for representing incoming signals.
- A way of representing structural information about these signals.

- Some definitions of a class of possible hypotheses about language structure.

- A method for establishing the meaning of each of these hypotheses in relation to each sentence.

- A method for selecting one of the many hypotheses dictated by some definitions of a class of possible hypotheses about language structure. This method also needs to be compatible with the given primary linguistic data.

In assuming that the primary linguistic data consist of signals made up of sentences, phrases, and words, Chomsky (1965) posits that the child must have an innate concept forming ability.

> Thus what is maintained, presumably, is that the child has an innate theory of potential structural descriptions that is sufficiently rich and fully developed so that he is able to determine, from a real situation in which a signal occurs, which structural descriptions may be appropriate to this signal, and also that he is able to do this in part in advance of any assumption as to the linguistic structure of this signal.
>
> (Chomsky, 1965, p. 32)

The implication is that the child possesses a *language-acquisition device* that translates a body of utterances into grammatical competence. The notion of grammar suggests a set of rules that turns ideas into sentences. This language acquisition device, or LAD as McNeil (1970) calls it, is a universal concept in that it serves to acquire any language because language shares a universal grammar. The same, however, cannot be said for the knowledge of language. For example, Chomsky (1986) points out that two people may share exactly the same knowledge of language but differ markedly in their ability to put this knowledge to use.

Elaborated and restricted codes

We have already suggested that there is an inextricable link between culture and the development of language. For example, individuals perceive the world as they do because they are primed to do so by the language of their culture to such an extent that language is seen as the mirror of society. In fact, at a macro-level Chaika (1982) boldly contends, 'there is no human society that does not depend upon, is not shaped by, and does not itself shape language' (p. 1). It could be argued that this still does not explain how or why individuals of the same culture speak differently. According to Bernstein (1964), the process and effect of socialisation would need to be understood at a micro-level of social interaction. For example, what in the environment is available for learning? What are the conditions that influence learning? What hinders or reinforces future learning? In order to grasp the concept of socialisation one would need to consider the basic difference between language and speech. From Bernstein's (1964) position there are two levels of language. The first level relates to its structure, for example the rules that regulate the use of language. The second level considers its vocabulary. Whereas structure serves to organise language, vocabulary conceptualises its meaning.

Language then represents the totality of options and the attendant rules for doing things with words. It symbolizes what can be done. Speech, on the other hand is constrained by the circumstances of the moment, by the dictate of a local social relation and so symbolizes not what can be done, but what is done with different degrees of frequency.

(Bernstein, 1964, p. 56)

Verbal language, in its totality of words and vocabularies, would seem to be regulated by an individual's social relationship. The implication is that what is said and how it is said depends on what is available in the social environment. For example, a word in English language may have more than one pronunciation depending on where the person is, Britain or United States of America. Similarly, two different words may have the same meaning, such as *boot* (British) and *trunk* (American), both are taken to mean luggage space in a car. Bernstein (1964) refers to this as 'linguistic code'. In relation to the language development of a child, Bernstein states that the identity of the social structure is transmitted to the child principally through this 'code'. 'From this point of view, every time the child speaks or listens, the social structure of which he is part of is reinforced and his social identity is constrained. The social structure becomes for the developing child his psychological reality by the shaping of his acts of speech' (Bernstein, 1964, p. 56). There is a controversial aspect to Bernstein's notion of linguistic code, and this relates to social class differences in language. Bernstein posits, although tenuously, that children who have access to different speech system by virtue of their status in social class structure may adopt quite different intellectual and social behaviour, and these may be associated with their psychological abilities (Bernstein, 1961). According to Sadovnik (2001), despite this controversy, crucial issues are raised about the relationships among the social division of labour, the family, and the school.

Bernstein (1964) identified two types of linguistic code, which he referred to as elaborated and restricted. Elaborated code allows individuals to select from a wide range of syntactic options, thus it may be difficult to predict their language organisation at any one time. Restricted code does not permit the luxury of options of wide range of syntactic alternatives (vocabulary of words are limited), this therefore makes prediction possible. The principal sentiment that one can deduce from the notions of elaborated and restricted codes is that the expression of language is much more explicit when one uses elaborated code in comparison to restricted code. However, the linguistic codes individuals use do not relate to what Bernstein calls 'innate intelligence', instead it is a question of sociological constraints exerted on them.

By attempting to explain the notion of language from a bio-psycho-social perspective we have considered each element (biological, psychological, and sociological) separately. However, this does not imply that these function in isolation. Indeed, it could be said that language mastery is dependent on all three elements. For example, the biological (including anatomical and physiological mechanisms) component needs to be fully functioning in order to receive, interpret, and send out information. Similarly, the information we send out depends on our attitude and perception of events. Moreover, every thing we see, hear, or say is influenced by our customs and habits, and these are individualised according to which group we belong, as well as what values we subscribe to.

Language and health care professionals

Health care language owes some of its origins to the tribal identities espoused by the rise of professional organisations, where membership had (and may still have) a unique way of communicating that affords its practitioners status as well as strengthening their position in society. Professional identity is enhanced by self-imposed regulation, for example, codes of professional conduct, where accountability and responsibility become enshrined in the language of any profession. It would be fair to say that each profession has its own culture defined by its own cognitive, affective, and behavioural orientations that are underpinned by their social heritage. It seems appropriate here to pause and consider Exercise 4.

EXERCISE 4

Reflect on your own particular professional discipline and define its culture. Take the word *culture* to mean *a way of life* that includes the ways its members behave and the value they subscribe to.

Describing one's own professional culture may not be as easy a task as it appears. One of the main difficulties as highlighted in Chapter 1 is that it is much more difficult to have an objective view of self from the *inside*, for example self-evaluating. As educationalists, we would find it easier to describe other professional cultures than our own. Perhaps an alternative would be to seek out what members of other professional cultures feel about your professional discipline. For example, it is not uncommon to hear the medical profession being described as patriarchal. 'During the industrial revolution, the medical profession established itself as the desired purveyor of care, delivered by male professionals for financial rewards. Cures of the professionally untrained healers and mid-wives (mainly women) were discredited' (Hall, 2005, p. 189). Contemporary attitude towards the medical profession has not deviated much from these previously held beliefs. Some would argue that once a profession becomes established, their language becomes part of their identity, and their influence depends on their position in society. For example, the medical profession probably holds one of the highest echelons in society and as such invites a certain degree of respect as well as subservience. The same could be said for other professional disciplines in that they would each shape their language and would in turn be shaped by it. For example, judiciary language displayed in a courtroom may only permit a person to give a *yes* or *no* answer to a question and no added information is deemed necessary at that point in time. Prosecutors tend to use a language that disempowers the person on trial in order to convince members of the jury of an individual's culpability. The use of language in health care can also be disempowering principally because practitioners are perceived as the voices of authority and to a greater extent whatever practitioners say, becomes the order of the day as exemplified by the following anecdotal account.

John, a middle aged man of African origin, was an inpatient at a mental health unit. Diagnosed as suffering from paranoid schizophrenia, John was observed to be symptom free and his discharge from the unit was imminent. However, John had been complaining of abdominal pain and was referred to Dr. Bob, a consultant physician who carried out a physical examination and related his findings to John's consultant psychiatrist but added his concern that John had threatened to kill him (Dr. Bob). Apparently, during the examination John was alleged to have said to Dr. Bob, *you will be punished for the way you are treating me*. Based on this new observation, John was not discharged but instead detained under section 3 of the Mental Health Act (1983) on the ground that he presented a danger to the public. John appealed against this detention order and at the hearing when asked why did he want to kill Dr. Bob, he replied, *it's not me who will punish the doctor, it's the Lord. The Lord is watching over me and protecting me from danger. The Lord will punish all those who are bad.* Members of the Review Tribunal concluded that although delusional John did not present a threat to the public. Common sense prevailed and John's compulsory detention was lifted and consequently discharged from the unit.

Interestingly, John's words were presumed to be of a delusional nature and no one even considered that it could be a true sentiment based on his cultural beliefs. The above scenario is a clear indication of how the misinterpretation of language can be to the detriment of patients. Dr. Bob should have been more attentive instead of perhaps allowing John's diagnosis to influence his judgement.

A general held belief is that health care professionals are quite good at using a language that only they can understand. Exercise 5 helps to focus your observation.

EXERCISE 5

At the next available opportunity, try and listen to any member of the health care team.

List any words or phrase used that you did not understand? How can the use of these words be justified?

One cannot deny the fact that health care language with its numerous terminologies can be very confusing, thus leading to misunderstanding. For example, Haffner (1992) gave an account of a 30-year-old pregnant woman from Mexico who was prescribed *Sitz* baths for immersion therapy for her swollen hands and arms. What the woman in fact did was to 'fill the bathtub with water and get in and sit down. Then she would stand up, sit down, stand up, sit down, stand up, sit down – for 20 minutes at a time' (Haffner, 1992, p. 258). This misunderstanding can be attributed to the fact that the doctor had presumed that the patient understood the prescription. The patient on her part perhaps interpreted the word *Sitz* to mean *sits* and it would make perfect sense that if prescribed *sits baths* it can only mean numerous *sits* in a bath.

Exercise 6 can be seen as a little test of your awareness of some health terminologies.

EXERCISE 6

Explain what you understand by each of the following words:

Toxic confusional state	Dysphagia	Aphonia	Angiography	Hemiplegia
Necrotic tissue	Apnoea	Aphasia	Myopia	Fistula
Incubation period	Neuralgia	Nephritis	Neonatal	Dyspepsia
Premorbid personality	Polyuria	Neuritis	Alopecia	Lumbar puncture

---

Perhaps some among us will find this exercise easier than others. The adage is *it is always easy when you know it*. For most members of the health care profession these words may form part of their common language. However, members of the lay public would perceive these as jargon, thus adding to the so-called mysticism to the health care profession. According to Ley (1988), some medical terminologies can and do lead to misunderstanding on patients' part. For example, some patients thought that a lumbar puncture was an operation to drain the lungs, while others thought incubation period was the length of stay the child would have to remain in bed. One could argue that perhaps Ley's findings are outdated and members of the public are now much more aware of medical terminologies. Based on our own experiences, we would argue that this is far from the case. However, our position is that language itself should not be held responsible for misunderstanding because it merely represents the symbol of communication. Instead, those who utter the words should take responsibility for making sure that listeners grasp their meanings. Health care languages can be perceived as disempowering especially when medical jargons become common parlance among health care professionals. For example, one of us came across the term 'TWOC' whilst marking an essay related to elimination, that is *getting rid of waste product*. No explanation was offered as to its meaning as the candidate must have assumed that the marker would know. The marker on his part struggled to see the relevance between *Taken With Out Consent* and care related to elimination unless of course the patient was involved in a TWOC offence. A sense of doubt was aroused on the part of the marker who felt disempowered by this lack of knowledge. We later discovered that the *TWOC* that this particular candidate was referring to was in fact an abbreviation for *Trial With Out Catheter*. *TWOC* may be well known to most in medical or surgical setting, however, one would not expect its use (and at that without any explanation) in an academic essay. The simple message is that knowledge should never be assumed. As health care professionals we owe it to patients to make clear our intention, thus reducing the risk of reinforcing the power differential (by virtue of knowledge, expertise, and status in society) that exists between health care professionals and patients.

It can't be emphasised enough that the expression of language, whether verbal or written, needs to be explicit and free from jargon. Defined as the technical phraseology of experts, jargon serves to limit the language and reading skills of lay people and will most likely lead to difficulty in comprehending both verbal and written language. This then raises the question of informed consent in health care. How informed can one be when presented with a language that does not form part of one's dictionary? Consider the word randomisation as an example, if you were not research aware, would you know what it means? In a study investigating physicians' explanation and parental understanding of randomisation in childhood leukaemia, Kodish et al. (2004) found that 50% of parents did not understand what it meant. Moreover, barriers to understanding were found to be especially pronounced among parents of racial minority and lower socioeconomic status (SES). Despite this, 84% of the children were enrolled in the study. One can only speculate that perhaps these parents felt the need to comply as a matter of obligation to those whom they believe hold the power to influence the care and treatment of their children. In 95% of cases a consent document was also presented to the parents (Kodish et al., 2004). According to Osborne (2001), informed consent documents are notoriously hard to read because most of these are written in a language beyond the comprehension of the ordinary person. According to Simon et al. (2006), practitioners on their part should use less technical language and shorter sentences to convey their messages. The way forward would seem to be clarity of expression, whether this is verbal or written.

Summary

The very essence of language is considered to rest with production and comprehension. From a biological perspective, these are found to be situated in the Broca and Wernicke's area, respectively. Evidence suggests that damage to these parts leads to inability to speak or understand depending on which area is affected. The development of language is dependent upon a certain level of maturation and growth, and this implies that its formation would need to be developed before the critical period elapsed, otherwise language becomes problematic, as was found to be the case with Genie. The psychological basis of language rests principally within cognitive development as espoused by Piaget, who further posits that the origin of thoughts and intellectual processes are firmly imbedded in a person's schema. From a sociological basis, language is seen to be situated outside the realm of inheritability, thus implying that one needs to learn to express language. Language is not only a tool for communicating thoughts but shapes it as well, as hypothesised by Sapir and Whorf. Moreover, the language a culture uses is believed to determine the way its members interpret information about the world and to a large extent helps to determine individuals' perception of reality. From a health perspective, language is the essence of care where its uses can serve to either empower or disempower depending on how this is communicated to patients.

References

Bernstein, B. B. (1961). Social class and linguistic development. In A. H. Halsey, J. Floud, and C. A. Anderson (eds.), *Education, Economy and Society*. New York: Free Press.

Bernstein, B. B. (1964). Elaborated and restricted codes: their social origins and some consequences. *American Anthropologist*, New Series, 66(6), Part 2: The ethnography of communication.

Bookheimer, S. (2002). Functional MRI of language: new approaches to understanding the cortical organization of semantic processing. *Annual Review of Neuroscience*, 25, 151–188.

Broca, P. P. (1861). Loss of speech, chronic softening and partial destruction of the anterior left lobe of the brain. *Bulletin De La Societe Anthropologique*, 2, 235–238. Available at http://psychclassics.yorku.ca/Broca/perte-e.htm.

Brown, R. (1976). Reference: In memorial tribute to Eric Lenneberg. *Cognition*, 4, 125–153.

Carroll, D. W. (1999). *Psychology of Language*. Pacific Grove: Brooks/Cole Publishing Company.

Chaika, E. (1982). *Language, the Social Mirror*. Rowley: Newbury House Publishers, Inc.

Cherry, C. (1966). *On Human Communication: A Review, a Survey, and a Criticism*. Cambridge and London: The M.I.T. Press.

Chomsky, N. (1965). *Aspects of the Theory of Syntax*. Cambridge: MIT Press.

Chomsky, N. (1975). *Reflections on Language*. New York: Pantheon.

Chomsky, N. (1986). *Knowledge of Language: Its Nature, Origin, and Use*. New York: Praeger Publishers Division.

Corballis, M. (1999). The gestural origins of language. *American Scientist*, 87(2), 138.

Curtiss, S. (1977). *Genie: A Psycholinguistic Study of a Modern-Day 'Wild Child.'* New York: Academic Press.

Dunbar, R. (1996). *Grooming, Gossip and the Evolution of Language*. Cambridge: Harvard University Press.

Elkind, D. and Flavell, J. H. (1969). *Studies in Cognitive Development: Essays in Honor of Jean Piaget*. New York: Oxford University Press.

Flege, J. E., Yeni-Komshian, G. H., and Liu, S. (1999). Age constraints on second-language acquisition. *Journal of Memory and Language*, 41, 78–104.

Geschwind, N. (1979). Specialization of the human brain. *Scientific American*, 241, 180–199.

Haffner, L. (1992). Translation is not enough: interpreting in a medical setting. In cross-cultural medicine-a decade later (Special Issue). *Western Journal of Medicine*, 157, 255–259.

Hakuta, K., Bialystok, E., and Wiley, E. (2003). Critical evidence: a test of the critical period hypothesis for second-language acquisition. *Psychological Science*, 14(1), 31–38.

Hall, P. (2005). Interprofessional teamwork: professional cultures as barriers. *Journal of Interprofessional Care*, 1 (Supplement), 188–196.

Harley, T. A. (2001). *The Psychology of Language: From Data to Theory*. Hove and New York: Psychology Press.

Hjelle, L. A. and Ziegler, D. J. (1992). *Personality Theories. Basic Assumptions, Research, and Applications.* New York: McGraw-Hill International Editions.

Hunt, J. Mcv. (1969). The impact and limitations of the giant of developmental psychology. In D. Elkind and J. H. Flavell (eds.), *Studies in Cognitive Development: Essays in Honor of Jean Piaget* (pp. 3–66). New York: Oxford University Press.

Inhelder, B. (1969). Memory and intelligence in the child. In D. Elkind and J. H. Flavell (eds.), *Studies in Cognitive Development: Essays in Honor of Jean Piaget* (pp. 337–364). New York: Oxford University Press.

Johnson, J. S. and Newport, E. L. (1989). Critical period effects in second language learning: the influence of maturational state on the acquisition of English as a second language. *Cognitive Psychology*, 21, 60–99.

Kay, P. and Kempton, W. (1984). What is the Sapir-Whorf hypothesis? *American Anthropologist*, New Series, 86(1), 65–79.

Kodish, E., Eder, M., Noll, R. B., Ruccione, K., et al. (2004). Communication of randomization in childhood leukaemia trials. *Journal of American Medical Association*, 291(4), 470–475.

Kohler, W. (1925). *The Mentality of Apes.* London: Harcourt.

Kolb, B. and Whishaw, I. Q. (2003). *Fundamentals of Human Neuropsychology.* New York: Worth Publishers.

Kring, A. M., Davison, G. C., Neale, J. M., and Johnson, S. L. (2007). Abnormal Psychology. New York: John Wiley and Sons, Inc.

Lenneberg, E. H. (1953). Cognition in Ethnolinguistics. *Language*, 29(4), 463–471.

Lenneberg, E. H. (1967). *The Biological Foundations of Language.* New York: Wiley.

Ley, P. (1988). *Communicating with Patients: Improving Communication, Satisfaction and Compliance.* London: Croom Helm.

McNeil, D. (1970). The acquisition of language: the study of developmental psycholinguistics. New York: Harper and Row.

Mental Health Act (1983). Chapter 20. London: HMSO.

O'Keefe, J. and Nadel, L. (1978). *The Hippocampus as a Cognitive Map.* Oxford: Oxford University Press.

Osborne, H. (2001). Health communications can affect the bottom line. *Patient Care Management*, 16(9), 9–10.

Porter-O'Grady, T. (2003). Language mistakes by interpreters blamed for medical errors. *Patient Care Management*, 19(3), 9.

Piaget, J. (1932). *The Moral Judgement of the Child.* London: Routledge & Kegan Paul.

Piaget, J. (1952). *The Origins of Intelligence in Children.* New York: International Universities Press.

Romanes, G. J. (1984). Origins of human faculty. In A. Lock and E. Fisher (eds.), *Language Development* (pp. 25–38). London: Croom Helm in association with The Open University.

Sadovnik, A. R. (2001). Basil Bernstein prospect. *The Quarterly Review of Comparative Education*, 31(4), 687–703.

Sapir, E. (1921). *Language: An Introduction to the Study of Speech.* New York: Harcourt, Brace, and Company.

Sapir, E. (1929). The status of linguistics as a science. *Language*, 5, 207–214.

Sapir, E. (1970). Language. In D. G. Mandelbaum (ed.), *Culture, Language and Personality: Selected Essays* (pp. 1–44). Berkeley: University of California Press.

Siegler, R. S. (1991). *Children's Thinking.* Englewood Cliff: Prentice Hall.

Simon, C. M., Zyzanski, S. J., Duran, E., Jimenez, X., and Kodish, E. D. (2006). Interpreter accuracy and informed consent among Spanish-speaking families with cancer. *Journal of Health Communication*, 11, 509–522.

Stein, J. F. (2003) Why did language develop? *International Journal of Pediatric Otorhinolaryngology*, 67 (Supplement 1), S131–S135.

Steven, G. (1999). Age at immigration and second language proficiency among foreign born adults. *Language in Society*, 28, 555–578.

Wernicke, C. (1874). *Der aphasische Symptomenconplex: Eine psychologische Studies auf anatomischer Basis* (The Aphasia Symptom-Complex: A Psychological Study on an Anatomical Basis). Breslau, Poland: Cohn and Weigert.

Whorf, B. L. (1956). Science and linguistics. In J. B. Carroll (ed.), *Language, Thought, and Reality: Selected Writings of Benjamin Lee Whorf* (pp. 207–219). Cambridge: MIT Press.

Intrapersonal Communication and Self-Awareness

Dev M. Rungapadiachy

OBJECTIVES

After reading this chapter you should be able to

■ Recognise and discuss the characteristics of intrapersonal communication.

■ Explore the influence of intrapersonal dynamics in relation to engaging with others in both a personal and professional capacity.

Introduction

It would be rather naïve to believe that communication is a simple act of exchanging information between speaker and listener. Communication is, as numerous writers have pointed out, a symbolic process of sharing meaning. However, as argued in Chapter 6, meaning of words is attributed by people and not conveyed by the word itself. There are principally two types of communication and these are at an INTRAPERSONAL and INTERPERSONAL level. Intrapersonal communication relates to the cognitive and emotive selves discussed in Chapter 1. During intrapersonal communication it would seem as if individuals are sending and receiving messages to and from themselves. This may sound a strange concept but in reality this is what in fact happens all the time. Intrapersonal elements such as thinking and feeling are the *energisers* of communication. These could be seen as the sources of communication and function on two levels: a conscious level where individuals are reasonably in tune with their thoughts and feeling during an interaction and an unconscious level where individuals are not aware of these dynamics. One can deduce from Chapter 1 that cognitive self serves to judge self, others, and self in relation to others. The emphasis here is on how the effectiveness of any interaction depends on one's attitude towards and perception of the other interactant and vice versa. Given its centrality in an individual's personality, values are determinants of attitudes as well as of behaviour. Therefore, no discussion on communication would be complete without an exploration of the notion of values and attitude.

Values

'A *value* is an enduring belief that a specific mode of conduct or end-state of existence is personally or socially preferable to an opposite or converse mode of conduct or end-state of existence' (Rokeach, 1973, p. 5). Values could be seen as standards that individuals subscribe to in pursuit of their life goals. For example, values allow people to discriminate and favour one particular ideology over another. Values are used in the way that individuals present themselves to others. Moreover, these serve as templates to make judgement on others. Values also help to persuade or influence others. Perhaps more importantly as far as communication is concerned, values can be used as excuses to rationalise our faux pas. For example, a hurtful comment to someone may be justified as *its for your own good*. Allport (1961) cites Spranger who defines six major value types and these are as follows.

- The theoretical value relates to an individual's search for *truth*. The dominant feature of theoretical value is that of being non-judgemental in relation to beauty or usefulness of objects, the primary goal is to observe and reason. A *thinking person* would aptly fit the theoretical value mould.

- The economic value by contrast deals with the usefulness of objects, for example, if something has no practical use then it has no worth to the individual who holds economic value. This implies that individuals who subscribe to the economic value are more materialistic in their outlook to life. As Allport (1961, p. 298) states, 'in his relations with people he is more likely to be interested in surpassing them in wealth than in dominating them (political value) or in serving them (social value)'. This is not too dissimilar to the notion of keeping up with the Jones's, but in this instance one is motivated to do better. People who hold economic value would choose commercial gains over any other values including beauty. For example, painting or drawings are only appreciated because of their price tags and not for their aesthetic characteristic.

- The aesthetic value relates to an individual's appreciation of beauty, for example, shapes, harmony, grace, symmetry, or fitness take priority in life. People who hold the aesthetic value are more likely to see 'truth as equivalent to beauty' (Allport, 1961, p. 298). Moreover, it is much more important to be charming than truthful. Similarly, beauty can cover the cracks.

- The social value focuses on the worth of people and anyone who subscribes to social value is perceived as kind, sympathetic, and unselfish. They could also be described as *people's people*. However, they are likely to consider those who hold theoretical, economic, and aesthetic values as cold and inhuman.

- The political value emphasises power as the most fundamental and universal of motives. Political value is seen as a common attribute for leaders in any professional discipline.

- The religious value deals with unity, for example, the person is mystical and tries to understand the universe as a whole. Religious experience is seen to contribute positively to life. It could be said that people who hold the religious value see the work of God in every event they encounter. Moreover, they seek to unite themselves with what could be seen as a spiritual reality by withdrawing from life through self-denial and meditation.

The description of these six types of values does not imply that there are six types of people. Far from it, this typology is only meant to show the values that people subscribe to. Moreover, it does not suggest that 'the types are necessarily good, or that they are ever found in their pure form. An ideal type is rather a "schema of comprehensibility" – a gauge by which we can tell how far a given person had gone in organizing his life by one, or more, of these basic schemes' (Allport, 1961, p. 297). Values hold varying intensity to each individual, for example, one person may be more attracted towards aesthetic value and less to economic value, whereas another may be more drawn to religious than theoretical value. To appreciate beauty over religion does not make a person inferior or superior to another. However, it is important to recognise and respect the value orientation of the other person. Exercise 1 focuses on awareness of self and others.

EXERCISE I

Reflect on your own sense of self and identify the values you subscribe to. Which one or two predominate the others?
Similarly, on observing the behaviour of friends, colleagues, or partners try and judge which value or values they subscribe to.

Attitudes

According to Allport (1935), attitude ascribes meaning to one's world, for example it determines what one will see, hear, think, and do. In fact, Allport (1935) defines attitude as a mental and neural state of readiness that is organised through experience and exerts a directive or dynamic influence upon an individual's response to all objects and situations with which it is related. Mental and neural state of readiness suggests that people's attitudes are not visible to one another but rather they serve to prepare them to behave in a certain way. However, attitudes are reflected in the way people behave (see Exercise 2).

EXERCISE 2

Someone you know (for example, a colleague) is walking towards you but as the person gets nearer to you he or she looks to the floor or ceiling thus avoiding your gaze. What can you infer by that person's behaviour in relation to his or her attitude towards you?

One could conclude from Exercise 2 one of the following. Firstly, that perhaps your colleague was preoccupied with something and at the point of encounter got distracted. Secondly, that your colleague was deliberate in his or her action, thus clearly indicating *no desire to acknowledge your presence*. In the second instance, one would not be far wrong to infer that your colleague's attitude towards you was negative. Attitude therefore can be said to have a directional property in that when it is positive it brings people closer towards their objects but when negative it has an escape or avoidance property. A negative attitude would thus involve any activity that is directed towards placing distance between the person and the object of one's attitude (McDavid & Harari, 1969). Attitude is also organised through experience in that people are not born with it instead they acquire their particular attitude principally by learning (direct or indirect experience, parental influence, group influence, as well as media influence). Exercise 3 might help to clarify the association of learning with attitude formation and attitude change.

EXERCISE 3

Give an example in each of the following whereby your attitude was acquired by
Learning
Parental influence
Group or peer influence
Media influence

Learning, through direct or indirect experience, contributes greatly to the formation of attitude. Two concepts within the realm of learning, that is, classical and operant conditioning (discussed in Chapter 4), explain clearly the dynamics of attitude formation or change. Classical conditioning as was discussed involves the repeated pairing of two stimuli until the presence of one evokes the expectation of the other. For example, if a person is repeatedly paired with negative attributes, sooner or later individuals' attitude towards him or her will be negative. Reflect on Exercise 1 in Chapter 6. It may well be that an individual's attitude towards a prostitute who is HIV positive is one of *you have asked for it; you got what you deserve*. By definition, the word *prostitute* has negative connotation such as unworthy use of self to earn a living or the hire of self for sexual intercourse and hence inherently negative. Operant conditioning, again as was discussed in Chapter 4, is based on Thorndike's (1911) law of effect, the essence of which is that if a particular attitude is rewarded it will most likely be exhibited, whereas an attitude that is detrimental or discomforting will be eradicated. Reflecting on Exercise 2 above, where our presence is not acknowledged chances are we will refuse to acknowledge the other person upon future encounter. A third type of learning is social learning (see Chapter 4) where perhaps the most influential figures are parents who represent role models for children. Right from an early age children learn from parents about social etiquettes and the rules of behaviour including, in some instances, what to think and how to feel in the presence of any particular object, event, or activity. Similarly, the influence of role models cannot be underestimated as Rungapadiachy (2003) found that for some of his participants (student nurses), it was quite easy to be influenced by the role models' attitudes. For example, 'you start good and you get sucked into either a ward regime that is poor or you just latch onto the members of staff and their ways of doing things' (p. 112).

Attitude exerts a directive or dynamic influence in that it makes people do what they do. In this instance, attitude is seen as a motivating factor, for example, our attitude towards a healthy lifestyle forces us to engage in keep fit exercises. However, it does not necessarily follow that an individual is always motivated towards positive behaviour, for example our liking for alcoholic drinks can lead to maladaptive behaviour. Similarly, a person's intense dislike for another may result in aggression.

Functions of attitude

Described as a functional construct, attitude serves to structure people's social world, thus facilitating decision-making (Russell, Blascovich, & Driscoll, 1992). The functions of attitude can be clustered into four principal themes: utilitarian or adaptive function, economy or knowledge function, expressive function, and ego-defensive function (McGuire, 1969).

- **Utilitarian or adaptive function**: It could be said that people hold a particular attitude for a specific reason (whether conscious or unconscious). Utilitarian, by definition, suggests an element of *making practical use of*, therefore if adopting a certain attitude helps people to fulfil their aims, the likelihood is they will maintain it. For example, if we want to be members of a *gang* then the expectation and possibly the prerequisite is that we would have to share the values of the *gang*. Similarly, excluding all other variables, if political party A promises to reduce taxes the likelihood is that we would vote for them more so than if political party B promises to raise taxes to pay for a cause that bears no relevance to us.

■ **Economy or knowledge function**: Rajecki (1990) believes that it is impossible for people to attend to every detail in their social life. This means that incoming information is clustered into broad categories and labels ascribed to them. Moreover, those very labels dictate their behaviour, for example, if some lecturers indiscriminately believe students to be an unmotivated group of people they will most likely dismiss students' plea for an *extension* to the submission deadline of their assignment. The word knowledge in this context does not imply fact or truth but simply serves to give meaning and understanding to the individual who holds this particular attitude (Oskamp, 1991).

■ **Expressive function**: Attitudes can often serve to reflect our social image as well as our self-concept. Basically, the attitude that we adopt allows others to know who we are and what we stand for. Campaigning against poverty or racial discrimination are two such examples.

■ **Ego-defensive function**: The notion of mental defence mechanism was introduced in Chapter 1 and as was highlighted involves an element of self-deception. For example, a rational explanation is found for an irrational behaviour (thinking, feeling, and acting). Oskamp (1991) believes that we all use defence mechanism to a certain extent, however, those 'who are insecure or feel inferior or who have deep internal conflicts' tend to use them more (p. 76).

Exercise 4 attempts to relate some of the functions of attitude to self.

EXERCISE 4

Given that we have already considered defence mechanism in some depth, reflect here on the three other functions of attitude (utilitarian or adaptive function, economy or knowledge function, and expressive function) and identify some personal examples.

Components of an attitude

There are essentially two perspectives on the structural nature of attitude; the first one, perceived as the old version (Oskamp, 1991), sees attitude as a single entity but with three components, for example, cognitive, affective, and behavioural. According to Rajecki (1990), the cognitive component refers to any information and knowledge (whether true or false) that people hold towards the object of their attitude. For example, BMW cars are better than Mercedes cars. This may or may not be true; however, for the person holding on to such a belief, this would be an accurate interpretation. The affective component relates to the feeling that is aroused by the object of one's attitude, for example, I like BMW cars. Affective component of an attitude can't be disputed because the person is merely expressing his or her likes or dislikes for the object of his or her attitude.

Behavioural component of attitude relates to the action that people take in relation to the object of their attitude. Hypothetically, given that money is not an issue, the person will most likely buy a BMW car instead of a Mercedes car. Based on the above explanation it would seem that there is clearly a relationship between affective, cognitive, and behavioural components of attitude. However, according to Oskamp (1991), regardless of how plausible the tri-componential perspective of attitude is, its empirical validity and usefulness remain in doubt. The question lies with the issue of consistency. For example, viewing attitude as a single entity would demand a greater degree of consistency between these three components. There are instances where this is far from the case as LaPierre's (1934) classic survey shows. LaPierre's survey lasted over a period of two years during which time he travelled extensively with a young Chinese student and his wife, both of whom were described as 'personable, charming, and quick to win the admiration and respect of those they had the opportunity to become intimate with' (LaPierre, 1934, p. 231). They visited and were served at numerous establishments and in only one out of the 251 instances were refused to be accommodated because of being Chinese. Six months later LaPierre sent a questionnaire with the following question, 'Will you accept members of the Chinese race as guests in your establishments?' to those hotels and restaurants. 128 responses were obtained from 81 restaurants and cafes and 47 hotels, auto-camps, and tourists homes. Interestingly, 92% of the former and 91% of the later said that they would not serve members of the Chinese race. One can conclude from this that behaviour is not always consistent with thought and/or feeling. LaPierre's experiment is not without its fair share of critiques (see, for example, Dillehay, 1973). However dated and whatever one may think of its methodological limitations, the fact remains that there are some inconsistencies between feeling, thinking, and action. Attitude also has a predictive property, for example, we may believe that our colleagues are untrustworthy, this makes us feel uncomfortable, therefore when we are in their company we always watch 'our backs'. However, it would be erroneous to believe this to be the state of affairs in every case. Clearly, there are instances where we may have negative thoughts and harbour negative feeling towards someone but we don't necessarily display negative behaviour towards that person. For example, no matter how negative we may feel towards our colleagues or how bad we may think of them, chances are we may not always act in a way that reflects our feeling and thinking as demonstrated by LaPierre (1934). Exercise 5 attempts to raise self-awareness.

EXERCISE 5

Recall one or two instances where there were some inconsistencies between your feeling, thinking, and action. Offer possible rationales.

Some of the reasons for the inconsistency between cognitive, affective, and behavioural components would include the prevailing situation in which individuals may find themselves where their behaviour is dictated, for example by the level of stress they are exposed to. As one of Rungapadiachy's (2003) participants explained, 'let's have no hassles, why should you go to work and get hassle? You know you're stressed out anyway. Let's make life easier and fit in with the rest of the staff team' (p. 112). Similarly, our behaviour is dictated by our professional code of conduct, for example, regardless of what we may feel and think of individuals who have committed atrocious acts of brutality, we could not refuse them health care services.

Inconsistencies or lack of correlation have lead to the theoretical view that these components (cognitive, affective, and behavioural) are entities in their own right. Fishbein and Ajzen (1975) posit that the meaning of the word 'attitude' should be confined to the affective component denoting the sentiment individuals hold for the object (feeling). The cognitive component is seen as the subjective evaluation of the characteristic of the object (belief). Similarly, behavioural component relates to the intended act (action). Viewing these components as separate entities explains why people don't always act on how they feel or what they think. The notion of 'lovable rogue' might be one way to show a mismatch between the cognitive, affective, and behavioural components. Rogue by definition implies a negative attribute and yet for some there also seems to be a pleasing quality about the person. It is not uncommon to hear comments such as, *he is a nice person but a horrible practitioner* or *he may not have the right attitude but his intention is good*. Perhaps the notion of cognitive dissonance may explain these dynamics.

According to Oskamp (1991), cognitive dissonance theory is a type of consistency theory whereby people try to maintain some congruence between their beliefs, attitudes, and behaviour. Once people are aware of this inconsistency they become uncomfortable and try to rid themselves of it. According to Festinger (1962), cognitions can exist in any individual in the following ways.

- **Irrelevance**: They bear no significance to one another, for example, cognition 1 'Jane is extremely attractive' and cognition 2 'it's Friday'. We would have difficulty in establishing the relationship between these two cognitions. We would conclude therefore that cognition 1 is irrelevant to cognition 2.

- **Consonance**: The implication is that there is a degree of agreement between two cognitions, for example, cognition 1 'Jane is extremely attractive' and cognition 2a 'Jane is a wonderful lecturer'. There is a clear relationship between cognition 1 and cognition 2a. Moreover, these two cognitions are aimed in the same direction in that these are positive attributes of Jane.

- **Dissonance**: Two cognitions conflict with one another, for example, cognition 1 'Jane is extremely attractive' and cognition 2b 'Jane is a thief'. These two cognitions are not consistent in fact, they would appear to conflict with one another.

According to Festinger (1962), when this happens, people are driven to try and reduce the dissonance into consonance. Therefore, we would need to change either of these two cognitions to face the same direction as the other. In changing cognition 1 to read 'Jane is ugly' we would achieve consonance with ease. Thus, Jane is an ugly thief. However, changing cognition 2b (Jane is a thief) would be much more difficult especially since Jane is extremely attractive. According to Festinger (1962), level of social support would help to reduce consonance. If others believe that Jane is extremely attractive then as Oskamp (1991, p. 243) states, 'a mild denial of reality' could come into play. Hence, Jane becomes a lovable rogue and to see her as a lovable rogue is much more acceptable than to see her for what she is, that is, extremely attractive but a thief. Moreover, *lovable rogue* is much more acceptable by society than a thief. Our attempt to reduce dissonance may have serious implication for health care in that 'some unprofessional behaviour will most likely remain unchallenged simply because the perpetrators happen to be socially attractive' (Rungapadiachy, 2003, p. 200).

Social cognition, social perception, and social judgement

According to Baron and Byrne (1997), social cognition is the manner in which people interpret, analyse, and remember information about the social world or as Fiske and Taylor (1991) state, 'the study of how people make sense of other people and themselves' (p. 1). Both social perception and social judgement form part of social cognition. Social perception can be described as the process whereby people form impressions of and make inferences about others. In another word, social perception leads to social judgement. According to Malebranche (1997), there is no sensation of external objects that does not involve one or more false judgements. Similarly, 'error is encountered only in the judgements we make that our sensations are in objects . . . Nothing is truer than that all visionaries see what they see; their error lies in their judgements that what they see really exists externally because they see it externally' (Lennon & Olscamp, 1997, p. 69). The implication therefore is that we may not always perceive the right picture or see people for who they really are. There are numerous explanations to the dynamic of social cognition and some of these include the notion of attribution, social categorisations and schema, attention and consciousness, and inferences. The intention in this chapter is to focus very briefly on each of these elements.

Attribution

Attribution is the process through which individuals seek to explain why they do what they do. According to Oskamp (1991), attribution is about making inferences about unobservable characteristics of other people, ourselves, objects, or events. There are essentially two types of attribution and these are dispositional and situational.

■ Dispositional attribution also known as internal attribution suggests that behaviour is ascribed to individuals themselves. For example, they may portray themselves as warm and approachable, it could be inferred, that this relates to their personality that is *they are nice people*. Going back to the example of the colleague who looks to the floor or ceiling in order to avoid our gaze, here one of our conclusions could be that this individual is an arrogant person. Arrogance is thus perceived as a trait of that person and hence dispositional attribution.

■ Situational attribution also known as external attribution implies that behaviour is the result of a person's reaction to the environment. For example, as your colleague was walking towards you, he or she was distracted by a loud noise coming from the ceiling and was thus unable to reciprocate your gaze. The cause of the behaviour would be seen to reside outside of the person and in particular a reaction to the loud noise. Your colleague's response would be attributed to the situation, hence situational or external attribution.

It could be said that the principal difference between dispositional and situational attribution is the fact that in the first instance there is personal causality. This means that behaviour and its consequence are purposeful, the responsibility of which lies with the person. According to Heider (1958), there are five levels of responsibility and these are association, causal responsibility, foreseeability, intentionality, and justification. Consider the following scenario.

You, together with other patients, are at your doctor's surgery when Homer rushed in wanting to speak to the doctor as a matter of urgency. Unfortunately, the doctor was busy with another patient. The receptionist kindly asked Homer to wait for five minutes. Homer became anxious, restless, impatient, and insisted that he can't wait any more as he has had enough of it all, at which point you intervene by saying this world would be a better place without people like him. Homer left the surgery saying that no one cares anymore. The following day Homer is found dead at his home having taken an overdose.

According to Fiske and Taylor (1991), association is the level of responsibility where 'a person is held accountable for an action with which he or she is not causally involved' (p. 26). Reflecting on the above scenario, the other patients could be accused of being responsible for Homer's death by association because it could be argued that they did not perceive Homer's desperate need for help (responsibility by association). However, you could be seen as having caused Homer's death by virtue of what you said that is, *the world would be better place without people like him*, and this could have tipped Homer over the edge, thus causing him to take the overdose. This level would be seen as causal responsibility that according to Fiske and Taylor (1991) occurs when a person performs an act that may not be intended nor anticipated, for example, you did not think or anticipate that Homer would kill himself. Moreover, it could be argued that as a health care professional you should have foreseen the outcome given Homer's mental health state. In this case, foreseeability would be present. This means that you should have been able to predict Homer's future course of action given his unstable mental health state. According to Oskamp (1991), where foreseeability is absent, an individual is less responsible. Similarly, if you had intended (intentionality) for your words *the world would be better place without people like him* to have the intended outcome then you would bear the greatest responsibility where you would not be able to justify (justification is absent) speaking to Homer the way you did. However, the doctor would be justified in not attending to Homer in view of the fact that he or she was in the middle of a consultation with another patient.

According to Fiske and Taylor (1991), there are six different theoretical perspectives that form part of the essence of attribution theory and these are Heider's analysis of common sense psychology (1958), Jones and Davis's analysis of correspondent inference theory (1965), Kelly's covariation and causal schema theory (1967), Schachter's theory of emotional lability (1959, 1964, 1971), Bem's self-perception (1967), and Weiner's attributional theory (1979). Only Jones and Davis's correspondent inference theory and Kelly's covariation theory will be discussed in this chapter. See Fiske and Taylor (1991) for a detailed explanation of the other perspectives on attribution theory.

Theory of correspondent inference

Jones and Davis (1965) formulated the correspondent inference theory that relates to the conditions whereby people make dispositional (internal) attributions of the behaviour of others. Let us suppose that you chose to come to City University for your study. The questions one would ask is why City University? Was it because you consider City to have a great nightlife? Was it because you believe City University has a good reputation? Or was it because you happen to live nearby, thus making it a cheaper option, as you would not have to seek student accommodation? Using the theory of correspondent inference, one should be able to identify your real motive for choosing to study at City University. According to Jones and Davis (1965), knowledge of people's traits and characteristics will lead us to understand and predict their behaviour. Moreover, the more intentional and consistent their behaviour, the more informed we become of why they behave as they do. Some of the factors that can increase correspondence of inferences include people's ability to freely choose their particular behaviour, social desirability, non-common effects, hedonistic relevance, and paternalism.

- **Behaviour needs to be voluntary**: As Pennington (2000) states, we cannot infer much about people's behaviour if they have little choice over what they do. The implication is that lack of options can only serve to predict that given the same situation we may all react in a similar way. For example, where one company has a monopoly of selling a particular utility the likelihood is that if we want that particular service then we will have to buy from that one company, as was previously the case in Great Britain with gas (British Gas) and telephone (British Telecom). It would be a pointless exercise to ask people why did they buy their gas from British Gas because we already know the answer and that is British Gas was the only supplier.

- **Social desirability**: Lack of social desirability of people's action is also significant in increasing correspondence of inference. For example, there may not be much to learn where a given behaviour is socially desirable because of our tendency to conform to the norm. Moreover, Baumeister and Leary (1995) found that the desire to please others often overrides people's own sense of self. Complying with the norm therefore is less revealing of a person's disposition other than their ability to be compliant. However, socially undesirable behaviour is more informative of a person's trait. 'When people are willing to break with norms or conventions to act in a certain way, one can be reasonably certain that their behaviour reflects their true beliefs because by so doing they are risking socially aversive consequences, such a rejection' (Fiske & Taylor, 1991, p. 29).

- **Non-common effects**: According to Jones and Davis (1965), when an action produces effects that differ from those that would have resulted from another action correspondent attribution is more likely. The principal sentiment underpinning non-common effect is the difference or uniqueness between two choices, which could be used to predict a person's choice. Let us suppose that you choose lecturer A instead of lecturer B for academic supervision. Each lecturer's traits are listed in Table 7.1 Given that there is a single non-common effect, one could infer that you chose lecturer A because you prefer to have someone who is an expert on your topic of study. However, too many non-common effects (different or unique effects) make it much more difficult to ascribe internal attribution for an individual preferred choices (see Table 7.2).

Table 7.1 Traits of two lecturers with a single non-common effect

Lecturer A	Lecturer B
Appears warm and approachable	Appears warm and approachable
Has a reputation to be sensitive to the needs of students	Has a reputation to be sensitive to the needs of students
An expert in your chosen topic of study	*Not an expert but is an experienced supervisor*
Has an open door policy for supervision	Has an open door policy for supervision

Table 7.2 Traits of two lecturers with three non-common effects

Lecturer A	Lecturer B
Appears warm and approachable	*Has a reputation to be too authoritarian*
Has a reputation to be sensitive to the needs of students	*Works according to the stated protocol*
An expert in your chosen topic of study	*Not an expert but is an experienced supervisor*
Has an open door policy for supervision	Has an open door policy for supervision

It becomes really difficult to identify one specific reason for your choice of lecturer because it could be any one of the first three characteristics and traits of lecturer A.

- **Hedonic relevance**: The concept of hedonic relevance is not dissimilar to the notion of apportioning blame or praise to someone as a result of a perceived weakness or strength in his or her character. According to Fiske and Taylor (1991), hedonic relevance refers to the effect an individual's behaviour has on the perceiver. For example, one of your lecturers gave you wrong advice and as a result you fail your assignment. It is most likely that you will perceive him or her as incompetent than if you had passed. One argument is that the greater hedonic relevance the more likely the perceiver is able to make a correspondence attribution.

- **Personalism**: This relates to the degree of intentionality such as *was the action deliberately aimed at the perceiver?* A common example is that of driver who deliberately increases speed to prevent you form overtaking. You are most likely to attribute a negative trait to him or her than you would if he or she had allowed you to pass.

Covariation theory of attribution

The formulation of the theory of covariation is credited to Kelly (1967) and differs from the theory of correspondent inferences in two ways. First, covariance relates to multiple events, whereas correspondence inference focuses on a single event. Second, covariance can apply to both dispositional and situational attributions, whereas correspondence inference is only implicated in dispositional attributions. According to Kelly (1967), 'the effect is attributed to that condition which is present when the effect is present and which is absent when the effect is absent' (p. 194). Let us analyse Exercise 2 one more time (a colleague is walking towards you but as the person gets nearer to you he or she looks to the floor or ceiling thus avoiding your gaze). Earlier, we were left with two options and these were that the avoidance of eye contact was (a) deliberate and (b) accidental. According to Kelly (1967), we can only confirm the accuracy of our attribution if an individual responds differentially (distinctiveness), consistently, in the same manner, and in agreement with a consensus of other people to the object or event.

- Distinctiveness can be established by asking whether or not this colleague is the only person who avoids our eye gaze? If the answer is yes, then we would say that there is a high distinctiveness about this person's behaviour, for example, avoiding eye gaze is unique to him or her.

- Consistency over time can be established by exploring its occurrence towards us over a period of time. For example, does the colleague nearly always exhibit this gaze avoidance behaviour? If yes, then there is a high consistency.

- Consensus can be established by asking if this colleague deliberately avoids eye gaze towards others as well. Again, if yes, there is a high consensus.

Our attribution of a trait is much more accurate when there is high distinctiveness, high consistency, and high consensus. In this instance, we could conclude that this colleague is *arrogant*. According to Oskamp (1991), accurate attribution could also be made where there is a low distinctiveness, high consistency, and low consensus. In this case, we could conclude other people avoid your eye gaze (low distinctiveness) almost all the time (high consistency), but this behaviour is only exhibited towards you and nobody else (low consensus). Therefore, we could attribute the problem to lie with you by presuming that all these people can't be wrong.

Errors and biases

'The psychologically naïve, unreflective person lives and acts under the silent assumption that he perceives other people in a factual, objective way. He is not aware of certain interpretative mechanisms at work within himself which distort and falsify his perception, observation, and interpretation of other people' (Ichheiser, 1970, p. 34). Here lies the justification for my emphasis on self-awareness as one way forward to enhancing care delivery. It is not the intention to group every health care professional into this category. However, there is a belief that not everyone is as self-aware as they think they are. Errors and biases fall into the realm of misperception and when events are perceived outside the context that which they appear, misinterpretation is most likely to occur. Using Heider's (1958) analogy, 'just as ambiguous words become more specifically defined when they are placed in sentences that give them a contextual setting the ambiguity of mediation events is reduced when stimulus of manifestations referring to distal stimulus are *embedded* in the total situation' (p. 37). The term embeddedness is taken to mean the integration of a stimulus (this can be anything from an event to an object) into its environment. Constructive embeddedness is associated with thinking, whereas destructive embeddedness is attributed to perception (Piaget, 1950). We could assume here that in constructive embeddedness (such as accurate interpretation) both stimulus and the situation at which they appear are taken as a *whole*. In other words, we have what would be called *objective reality*. Similarly, with destructive embeddedness, events or objects are seen in isolation (such as outside the context at which they occur). Here, therefore, we deny, what Piaget (1950) calls, the possibility of objectivity, the outcome, thus, is misperception. According to Heider (1958), it is the surrounding situation that enables individuals to establish the motivations and intentions for a particular behaviour. As far as human relationships are concerned, Ichheiser (1970) believes that two crucial factors are responsible for misinterpretation and misunderstanding of other people's personality. Personality is taken to mean who we are.

1. We are different but in what sense? For example, how are we different, why are we different, and to what extent are we different?

2. We all act and react in a framework of different situations but we are unaware of the full implications of this part of the nature of human relations.

As Ichheiser (1970) states, 'we have the tendency to consider a partial structure of personality which happens to be visible to us as if this partial structure were the total personality itself' (p. 51). This phenomenon is seen as the tendency to overestimate personality unity. Ichheiser (1970) argues that unconscious interpretation plays the most significant role in how individuals see others because it operates on a much deeper level of social perception than conscious interpretation. For example, conscious interpretation would require the person to be much more cognisant of certain facts as well as other mental processes. Unconscious interpretations by definition suggest that individuals are not aware of their operations. For all intents and purposes, we think we have got it right until faced with contradictory evidence. For example, we may have always put someone on a pedestal until we realise that this person has deceived us all along. Similarly, we may have always had a negative impression of some people until we discover what they are truly like. According to Ichheiser, people are not confronted with the individuals themselves but instead their image that must have been distorted by mechanisms which operate on an unconscious level within our mind. This can be validated by such experiences as having preconceptions of people whom we have not even met. For example, we may have heard someone speaking over the phone and never actually met him or her face to face but this does not stop us from formulating a picture in our heads as to what the person looks like. As Ichheiser says that faced with reality, we are surprised and it is not uncommon to hear ourselves thinking *I expected you to be different* or words to that effect.

Kelly (1967) posits that attribution processes are no different to any other perceptual and cognitive system in that these are subject to error. Moreover, attribution errors can occur because of the following.

- **The relevant situation is ignored**: The implication here is that we tend to attach too much significance to people's behaviour and its effects and too little attention is paid to its situational context. This, according to Heider (1958), is because behaviour 'has such salient properties it tends to engulf the total field rather than be confined to its proper position as a local stimulus whose interpretation requires the additional data of a surrounding field . . .' (p. 54). The notion of fundamental attribution error would seem to function under similar principles. Fundamental attribution error can be described as the attribution of someone's behaviour to his or her dispositional qualities, thus totally ignoring any situational factor. This implies that an individual is deemed to be wholly responsible for the exhibited behaviour. Interestingly, however, fundamental attribution error is only related to the behaviour of others and not to one's own. According to Fiske and Taylor (1991), fundamental attribution error occurs because the dominant aspect of a person's behaviour is what he or she does, for example, the person engages in numerous activities that attract attention. Background factors as well as rationale for behaviour pale into insignificance. Therefore, we perceive the foreground while totally ignoring the background.

- **Egocentric assumptions are made**: According to Heider (1958), we have a tendency to make attribution based on our own needs or wishes when faced with insufficient information. For example, if I like something, others will like it too and to some extent we come to expect it. I might make my wife a cup of tea based on how I like my tea.

From Ichheiser's (1970) perspective, 'we often deceive ourselves into believing that we interpret and evaluate other people according to the merits of their personal characteristics' (p. 56). The truth, however, is that we evaluate others (and to some extent ourselves) by the consequence of their actions, for example according to success or failure. This makes our evaluation and judgement of others conditional.

Actor–observer effect

The phenomenon of actor–observer effect as related to fundamental attribution effect can be best explained via Exercise 6.

EXERCISE 6

Think of the last time you encountered someone whom you would describe as hostile. Make a list of the traits and characteristics that led you to this label. Now take a closer look at these traits and characteristics. Try and recall if at any time in the past you have exhibited these characteristics.

Perhaps it would be fair to say that it is highly unlikely that we would see ourselves as hostile regardless of the fact that we may have exhibited hostile behaviour. The answer would seem to lie with the phenomenon of actor–observer effect, which can be described as the tendency to ascribe the behaviour of others to dispositional factors (when people make mistakes they are stupid), whereas our own behaviour is attributed to situational factors (if we make a mistake it would be because we were distracted). One possible explanation for the actor–observer effect is lack of self-awareness. Moreover, it would be erroneous to believe that actor–observer effect is a conscious act as Fiske and Taylor (1991) explain, 'as an actor, one literally cannot see one's self-behaving, and so one's own behaviour or activity is not particularly salient. Rather, the situational forces impinging on one's behaviour are salient, and so they are perceived as exerting a causal influence' (p. 73). This is not too dissimilar to the analogy of *viewing the world and its occupants with a different pair of glasses than the ones we use to view ourselves*. A number of issues related to self are addressed in Chapter 1. The ensuing discussion will focus on the notion of impression formation.

Impression formation

In order to understand the notion of impression formation, we would need to revisit the word schema introduced in Chapter 6 where schema was described as a cognitive structure that serves to help individuals to perceive, organise, process, and use information about the world. In simple terms schema is 'an abstract, general expectation about how some part of the world operates, built up on the basis of our own past experience with specific examples' (Oskamp, 1991, p. 31). Schema, in particular social schema, can be seen as the foundation for impression formation. There are at least four types of social schemas and these are person schema, self-schema, role schema, and event schema (Fiske & Taylor, 1991). Moreover, they all have similar purposes in that they impact on the assimilation and interpretation of 'new information, memory for old information, and inferences about missing information' (Fiske & Taylor, 1991, pp. 117–118).

- Person schemas can be described as those traits and characteristics that individuals use in order to understand types of people or specific individuals. Zebrowitz (1990) sees person schemas as the knowledge about personality that relates to the psychological grouping of people. For example, we may see people as extroverts or introverts. In simple terms, it could be said that person schema is more like a template that individuals use to make sense of other people. Similarly, a schema that relates to a particular social group could be seen as a stereotype, which can be described as 'a generalization about a group of people in which identical characteristics are assigned to virtually all members of the group, regardless of actual variation among the members' (Aronson, Wilson, & Akert, 1997, p. 479). According to Allport (1954), a stereotype is an exaggerated belief associated with a category and serves to justify people's conduct in relation to that particular category. However, one should not confuse stereotype with categorisation, because as Allport (1954) states, 'a stereotype is not identical with a category; it is rather a fixed idea that accompanies the category' (p. 191). A stereotype can be favourable (Italian men are romantic) or unfavourable (Black people are lazy). Stereotypes are resistant to change even when confronted with factual information.

- Self-schemas can be described as an organised knowledge of self (see 'Self-Concept' in Chapter 1). For example, people may have a clear picture of some of their traits. According to Fiske and Taylor (1991), 'people who hold self-schemas for a particular domain, whether shyness, independence, or creativity, for example, consider the domain to be personally important and typically have well-developed conceptions of themselves in these domains' (p. 183). This could mean that the level of importance one places on a domain may dictate the level of awareness of that particular domain.

- Role schemas clearly relate to an expected set of behaviours from people depending on their position in society. According to Fiske and Taylor (1991), role schema is 'the cognitive structure that organizes one's knowledge about those appropriate behaviours' (p. 119). For example, as a health care professional, one is expected to behave in a caring way towards those in need of health services. An individual may have numerous roles, for example, son/daughter, mother/father, health care practitioner, lecturer, and so on.

Each of these roles has a prescribed set of behaviour. Moreover, roles can be ascribed (by virtue of birth, for example son and daughter) and achieved (by virtue of work and effort such as lecturer or doctor).

- Event schemas also known as scripts relate to the knowledge about the procedures associated with familiar social situations, for example one is aware of what goes on at a football game, wedding, funeral, pop concert, and so on. The implication is that one is aware of the sequence of events that takes place at these social situations. Obviously, some event schemas are contingent upon an individual's culture. For example, while the sequence of events at a football game or pop concert may be common to every culture, funerals and weddings are not.

Self-serving bias and self-centred bias

Self-serving bias can be described as 'the tendency to take credit for success and deny responsibility for failure' (Fiske & Taylor, 1991, p. 78). For example, when students do well in their assignments we pride ourselves for being good lecturers but when students do poorly we think of them in terms of lacking cognitive ability to grasp concepts. Moreover, individuals would not like to think of themselves as incompetent. Self-serving biases provide some comfort in that individuals see themselves free of responsibility for failures, thus protecting their own self-esteem. According to Fiske and Taylor (1991), it is always desirable to have others think of us as competent, thus leaving us free to perform as we wish, for example we could perform well or we could perform badly and this would not affect other people's perception of us. However, to be perceived as incompetent can be, what Fiske and Taylor (1991) call, 'constraining'. A constraining portrayal of self is seen as limiting because it forces an individual to 'go to great lengths to keep both the self and others from making low ability attribution' (Fiske & Taylor, 1991, p.235). It would be erroneous to generalise the notion of self-serving bias to apply to every individual in every situation. As Pennington (2000) points out that some people do show modesty when being praised for some heroic deed and in some cases it is not uncommon to hear such statement as *well, this would not have been possible had it not been for my team.* Interestingly, however, Miller and Schlenker (1985) found 'that group members are cognizant of the audiences which will encounter their attributions, and that they regulate their reports accordingly' (p. 88). For example, in describing their responsibility Miller and Schlenker's (1985) participants were described as egotistical in private but not in public, thus concluding that their participants 'were clearly sensitive to the interpersonal implications of their attributions, displaying less egotism under public conditions' (p. 85).

The notion of self-centred bias (also known as egocentric bias) can be described as the taking of credit for more than one's share of responsibility for a task that is performed by two or more people. This is not dissimilar to a person's belief that he or she works harder than everyone else. According to Ross and Sicoly (1979), there are at least four explanations as to why self-centred bias may occur and these are as follows.

1. **Selective encoding and storage**: We are basically more aware of the things that we do than what other people do. The implication is that our own thoughts and actions may serve to distract us from noticing how much others have contributed.

2. **Differential retrieval**: The emphasis here is on recalling, 'how much did I contribute?' (Ross & Sicoly, 1979, p. 323). This implies that an individual tends to attempt to recall principally his or her own contribution, thus ignoring the contribution of the other person.

3. **Informational disparities**: We may not always recognise the extent to which the other person has contributed especially since their contribution took place in our absence. Ross and Sicoly (1979) posit that we each have greater access to our own individual internal states and thoughts than others would have of us.

4. **Motivational influences**: One's own self-esteem would seem to be an important issue in mediating self-centred bias. For example, thinking about our own input may serve to enhance our own sense of self.

Summary

Intrapersonal elements, such as thinking and feeling, can be described as the very essence of communication where values, beliefs, and attitudes influence interactions between individuals. These are said to function on both a conscious and unconscious level. Intrapersonal communication necessitates the need for self-awareness in order to decrease unconscious level of functioning, thus increasing knowledge of self and of others. Described as the way people make sense of their world, social cognition consists of social perception in the shape of impression formation that is influenced by social judgement. For a variety of reason discussed, the impression and judgement individuals make of themselves and of one another are not always accurate. Theories of correspondent inference and covariation attempt to explain an individual's intrapersonal dynamics. Moreover, errors and biases are believed to play a significant role in interpersonal communication.

References

Allport, G. W. (1935). Attitudes. In C. Murchison (ed.), *Handbook of Social Psychology* (pp. 798–844). Worcester: Clark University Press.

Allport, G. W. (1954). *The Nature of Prejudice*. Cambridge: Addison-Wesley Publishing Company, Inc.

Allport, G. W. (1961). *Pattern and Growth in Personality*. New York: Holt, Rinehart, and Winston.

Aronson, E., Wilson, T. D., and Akert, R. M. (1997). *Social Psychology*. New York: Longman.

Baron, R. A. and Byrne, D. (1997). *Social Psychology* (8th edition). Boston: Allyn and Bacon.

Baumeister, R. F. and Leary, M. R. (1995). The need to belong: desire for interpersonal attachments as a fundamental human motivation. *Psychological Bulletin*, 117, 491–529.

Bem, D. J. (1967). Self-perception: an alternative interpretation of cognitive dissonance phenomena. *Psychological Review*, 74, 183–200.

Dillehay, R. C. (1973). On the irrelevance of the classical negative evidence concerning the effect of attitudes on behaviour. *American Psychologist*, 28, 887–891.

Festinger, L. (1962). *A Theory of Cognitive Dissonance*. Stanford: Stanford University Press.

Fishbein, M. and Ajzen, I. (1975). *Belief, Attitude, Intention, and Behaviour: An Introduction to Theory and Research*. Reading: Addison-Wesley.

Fiske, S. T. and Taylor, S. E. (1991). *Social Cognition*. New York: McGraw-Hill, Inc.

Heider, F. (1958). *The Psychology of Interpersonal Relation*. New York: Wiley.

Ichheiser, G. (1970). *Appearances and Realities*. San Francisco: Jossey-Bass.

Jones, E. E. and Davis, K. E. (1965). From acts to dispositions: the attribution process in person perception. In L. Berkowitz (ed.), *Advances in Experimental Social Psychology* (Vol. 2, pp. 219–226). New York: Academic Press.

Kelly, H. H. (1967). Attribution theory in social psychology. In D. Levine (ed.), *Nebraska Symposium on Motivation* (Vol. 15, pp. 192–238). Lincoln: University of Nebraska Press.

LaPierre, R. T. (1934). Attitudes vs. actions. *Social Forces*, 13, 230–237.

Lennon, T. M. and Olscamp, P. J. (1997). *Malebranche: The Search After Truth*. Cambridge, New York, and Melbourne: Cambridge University Press.

Malebranche, N. (1997). *The Search After Truth*. Translated and edited by Thomas M. Lennon and Paul J. Olscamp. Cambridge, New York, and Melbourne: Cambridge University Press.

McDavid, J. W. and Harari, H. (1969). *Social Psychology: Individuals, Groups, Societies*. New York, Evanston, and London: Harper and Row and John Weatherhill, Inc.

McGuire, W. J. (1969). The nature of attitudes and attitude change. In G. Lindzey and E. Aronson (eds.), *Handbook of Social Psychology* (pp. 233–346). (Vol. 2, 3rd edition). New York: Random House.

Miller, R. S. and Schlenker, B. R. (1985). Egotism in group members: public and private attributions of responsibility for group performances. *Social Psychology Quarterly*, 48, 85–89.

Oskamp, S. (1991). *Attitudes and Opinions*. Englewood Cliffs: Prentice Hall.

Pennington, D. C. (2000). *Social Cognition*. London: Routledge.

Piaget, J. (1950). *The Psychology of Intelligence*. New York: Harcourt-Brace.

Rajecki, D. W. (1990). *Attitudes*. Sunderland: Sinauer Associates.

Rokeach, M. (1973). *The Nature of Human Values*. New York: The Free Press and London: Collier Macmillan Publishers.

Ross, M. and Sicoly, F. (1979). Egocentric biases in availability and attribution. *Journal of Personality and Social Psychology*, 37, 322–337.

Rungapadiachy, D. M. (2003). *The Role of the Mental Health Nurse: A Comparison of the Perceptions of Mental Health Nurses at Three Levels of Experience (Pre-Post Registration, and Experienced Mental Health Nurses)*. Unpublished Thesis. University of Leeds, Leeds.

Russell, H. F., Blascovich, J., and Driscoll, D M. (1992). On the functional value of attitudes: the influence of accessible attitudes on the ease and quality of decision making. *Personality and Social Psychology Bulletin*, 18, 388–401.

Schachter, S. (1959). *The Psychology of Affiliation*. Palo Alto: Stanford University Press.

Schachter, S. (1964). The interaction of cognitive and physiological determinants of emotional state. In L. Berkowitz (ed.), *Advances in Experimental Social Psychology* (Vol. 1, pp. 49–82). New York: Academic Press.

Schachter, S. (1971). *Emotion, Obesity, and Crime*. New York: Academic Press.

Thorndike, E. L. (1911). *Animal Intelligent: Experimental Studies*. New York: Macmillan Press.

Weiner, B. (1979). A theory of motivation for some classroom experiences. *Journal of Educational Psychology*, 71, 3–25.

Zebrowitz, L. A. (1990). *Social Perception*. Milton Keynes: Open University Press.

Interpersonal Communication and Interpersonal Skills

8

Jack Morris and Dev M. Rungapadiachy

After reading this chapter you should be able to

▪ Recognise and discuss the characteristics of interpersonal communication.

▪ Evaluate the significance of interpersonal communication in relation to your own practice.

Introduction

Some would argue that communication is the very essence of human interaction whereby individuals send messages to one another. The implication is that communication is a continuous and never-ending process with no beginning. For example, the minute one walks into a room, one is sending and receiving messages. However, the sending of messages could be conscious and deliberate or unconscious and unintentional. In the first instance, the purpose of these messages is meant to initiate some sort of a response, whereas in the second instance no response is intended but there may be an impact. Often described as a complex and dynamic process, communication involves numerous 'self-variables' (discussed as intrapersonal factors in Chapter 7) on the part of both SENDER and RECEIVER who serve to influence these messages, for example, self-esteem, self-efficacy, gender, motivation, self-perception, and perception of others. It would therefore be a myth to believe that communication is a simple act of sending and receiving messages. Communication in its truest form would suggest that messages are sent and received in the manner in which these are intended or to put it simply *if we are able to capture the sentiments of your message and respond appropriately then and only then we would have communicated with you.* Adler and Rodman (2003) phrase it differently by stating that 'communication isn't a series of incidents pasted together like photographs in a scrapbook; instead, it is more like a motion picture in which the meaning comes from the unfolding of an interrelated series of images' (p. 3). This chapter focuses on interpersonal communication and the skills involved.

What is interpersonal communication?

According to Bochner (1985), interpersonal communication is 'a vague, fragmented, and loosely defined subject that intersects all the behavioural, social, and cultural sciences' (p. 27). The implication is that interpersonal communication is a much more complicated concept to fit in one global perspective. However, Adler and Rodman (2003) believe that interpersonal communication needs to be viewed not only in context of the number of people involved but essentially by the quality of the interaction. This means that we may need to go some way beyond person-to-person(s) interaction in order to fulfil the criteria for an accurate interpretation of interpersonal communication. For example, one would hardly call any interaction between a lecturer and his or her students an interpersonal communication. The same could be said for an interaction between a sales person and his or her potential customer. In fact, this latter type of interaction would seem to be a better fit in what has been described as impersonal communication (Adler & Rodman, 2003). An obvious starting point to understanding the notion of interpersonal communication is with person perception. This would imply that unless we are quite clear in our mind how we perceive the notion of person the meaning of interpersonal communication would remain vague, fragmented, and possibly elusive. Berenson (1981) posits that there are two ways to look at a person, for example, 'seeing a person as a person and seeing the person as the particular kind of person he is' (p. 73). One could deduce that generally seeing a person as a person lends itself to being somewhat impersonal in that seeing person A as a person is no different to seeing person B as a person because although we come in different shapes, sizes, and colour we are essentially anatomically and physiologically similar. However, seeing person A as a particular kind of person is a different issue altogether and would require the perceiver to restructure his or her general schema of person, thus adding a certain quality to that perception. Implicit within this type of perception is the notion of *personal*, or to put it simply, we are adding a sense of uniqueness to that person, thus *individuating* him or her. This sense of uniqueness can only be achieved if we understand the person at a deeper level that requires us to 'stand in some kind of personal relationship to him thus being in a position to have personal insights, to have direct experience of how his thoughts and feelings find expression in reciprocal relationships' (Berenson, 1981, p. 78). For example, the schema of someone's wife or husband as *a person* is bound to be qualitatively different to the schema of a passer-by as a person. Wife or husband therefore would fit in the category of *a particular kind of person* and our interaction would truly fit in the context of interpersonal communication.

Reflecting on the above discussion, it becomes clear that for any interaction to be confidently placed in the realm of interpersonal communication it must satisfy the following criteria; a person needs to be seen as unique as in *a particular kind of person* and there would need to be some element of closeness between the interactants as well as some reciprocal relationship. A word of caution about the notion of reciprocation is that according to Duck (1999), reciprocity in communication is seen as a somewhat superficial relationship between the interactants. For example, in a relationship reciprocity can be seen more as an obligation in that there is an implicit need to respond with a similar type of behaviour. For example, someone invites us for a meal and we try and find the earliest opportunity to return the gesture. Reciprocity in this context feels like *turn taking* and 'the more superficial the relationship, the more people keep count of whose turn it is to do the behaviour next' (Duck, 1999, p. 42). In this sense, therefore, reciprocity would seem more of a strategy that one would adopt during impersonal communication. However, where there is a much more meaningful relationship between two individuals reciprocity would serve to enhance interpersonal communication. Perhaps, a more appropriate dynamic would be that of Duck's (1999) notion of complementarity. Complementarity is different to reciprocity in that here people's needs are taken into account and is less superficial. For example, you may ask a friend to lend you a book and your friend would comply. However, there is no expectation that you have to do the same thing in return. According to Duck (1999), complementarity behaviour allows individuals to consider each other's needs, thus adding more depth to their relationship. On a final note about the definition of interpersonal communication, Adler and Rodman (2003) state that interpersonal communication takes place when 'people treat one another as unique individuals, regardless of the context in which the interaction occurs or the number of people involved' (pp. 184–185). The emphasis is very much on the uniqueness of the person. Exercise 1 is an attempt to clarify the notions of impersonal and interpersonal communication.

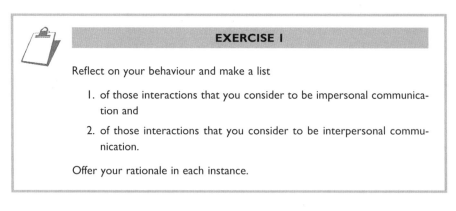

EXERCISE 1

Reflect on your behaviour and make a list

1. of those interactions that you consider to be impersonal communication and

2. of those interactions that you consider to be interpersonal communication.

Offer your rationale in each instance.

The goal of interpersonal communication

It could be argued that if interpersonal communication has a fundamental goal then it follows that there has to be an interpersonal need. Recognising that people need people Schutz (1966) posed the question, 'in what ways do people need people'? Before attempting to answer this question consider Exercise 2.

EXERCISE 2

Consider the time when you have been treated in an impersonal way (contrary to how it should have been). How did this make you feel?

Given that interpersonal communication serves to make the uniqueness of an individual more visible, what are the benefits of being perceived as unique?

It could be said that perhaps the principal goal of interpersonal communication is the recognition and validation of one's *sense of being* in a meaningful way, in other words, to be accepted and prized by others. This can be clarified further by exploring two of Maslow's (1968) hierarchy of needs: love and belongingness, and esteem needs. The implication is that provided our physiological needs and safety needs are satisfied (partly or wholly), we then would develop a hunger for interpersonal relationship because only other people can satisfy our needs for love and belongingness, and esteem, clearly implying that people do need people. We are basically dependent on others for survival.[1] Love and belongingness as well as esteem needs are clustered in what Maslow (1968) calls deficiency needs (or motives) to suggest that their satisfaction or presence would prevent illness. Moreover, Maslow argues that basic needs are found to be inactive or functionally absent in the healthy person. It could be said, however, that healthy people would need to have a regular supply of these deficiency needs in order not to feel depleted, otherwise it could be a case of too many inappropriate impersonal communication that could lead to a lower sense of self. This was found to be the case in a small qualitative study conducted by Murira et al. (2003), where communication patterns between health care providers and their clients at an antenatal clinic in Zimbabwe revealed a negative effect on these women's personal and unique identity. Impersonal language such as 'the woman with multiple pregnancies', 'the woman referred from X clinic', 'the woman in a red dress', and 'the short woman' was reported to be typical of midwives' behaviour (Murira et al., 2003, p. 86). Maslow (1999) would argue that by definition, health care must be interpersonal. Emphasis is placed on the *must* because one of the defining characteristics of people who seek health care points to some deficiencies of their basic needs and 'because this is so, a basic necessity for cure is supplying what has been lacking or making it possible for the patient to do this himself' (Maslow, 1999, p. 43). To this end, the interaction between health care professionals and patients could be described as a dependency relationship hence, not a reciprocal one. The implication is that, health care professionals' behaviour affects patients but is not affected by patients. Exercise 3 aims to raise awareness of the use of language and its implication on patients.

EXERCISE 3

Reflect on your particular health care environment, recall and list any language used that may have contributed to unwarranted impersonal communication.

Imagine how it must feel to be treated in an impersonal manner.

It would be erroneous to believe that lack of interpersonal communication in health care is isolated to one specific country. It is not uncommon to hear such words or phrases as the paranoid schizophrenic, the demented, the abused, the casualty, the victim, and the catheter.

Three fundamental interpersonal needs

According to Schutz (1966, p. 1), 'people need people for three kinds of relations' and these are inclusion, control, and affection. Each of these needs can be recognised by three particular types of behaviour and these are as follows.

1. Deficient means that the individual does not attempt to search for inclusion, control, and affection.

2. Excessive suggests that the individual is constantly trying to search for inclusion, control, and affection.

3. Ideal relates to an individual who is quite content in that the need for inclusion, control, and affection are satisfied.

The need for inclusion is not too dissimilar to Maslow's (1999) need for love and belongingness, and esteem need. The implication is that inherent to being human, every individual has a need to establish and maintain what Schutz (1966) calls 'a satisfactory relation with people with respect to interaction and association' (p. 18). Satisfactory relation, however, has two dimensions: psychological and emotional. Being psychologically comfortable in relationships would seem to be individually defined in that this ranges from the need to initiate interaction with all people to the need of not to initiate interaction with anyone. One could take this to mean that some people prefer to be undersocial other people prefer to be oversocial and still others are quite content being social. Hayes (1991) sums the notion of inclusion as the 'need to be with people and to be alone, to have enough contact to avoid loneliness and enough aloneness to avoid enmeshment and enjoy solitude' (p. 255).

People who do not make an attempt to search for inclusion are described as *undersocial*. They are perceived as introverts and would thus consciously establish and maintain distances between self and others. According to Schutz (1966), one of the rationales for such behaviour is an unconscious desire for others to pay them attention. However, their biggest fears are feelings of rejection. This could imply that being undersocial could be a defence mechanism (see Chapter 1) employed by these type individuals in order to safeguard their psychological and emotional vulnerability. The sentiments of those people could be captured by 'no one is interested in me, so I'm not going to risk being ignored. I'll stay away from people and get along by myself' (Schutz, 1966, p. 26). People who are *oversocial* on the other hand exhibit a complete opposite behaviour. For example, they would constantly seek other people's company because they can't bear to be on their own. These types of individual could be described as extraverts, reflecting a behaviour that is designed to focus attention on themselves and have other people noticing them. A third type of inclusion is characterised by people who have no problem with the need to be *in* or *out*. They are described as *social* because they feel comfortable with or without the company of other people. There is no desperate need on their part to either seek or avoid the company of other people. Exercise 4 aims to situate the type of inclusion within self.

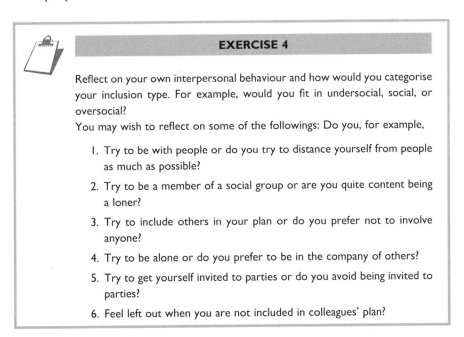

EXERCISE 4

Reflect on your own interpersonal behaviour and how would you categorise your inclusion type. For example, would you fit in undersocial, social, or oversocial?

You may wish to reflect on some of the followings: Do you, for example,

1. Try to be with people or do you try to distance yourself from people as much as possible?

2. Try to be a member of a social group or are you quite content being a loner?

3. Try to include others in your plan or do you prefer not to involve anyone?

4. Try to be alone or do you prefer to be in the company of others?

5. Try to get yourself invited to parties or do you avoid being invited to parties?

6. Feel left out when you are not included in colleagues' plan?

According to Schutz (1966), the interpersonal need for control can be seen as 'the need to establish and maintain a satisfactory relation with people with respect to control and power' (p. 18). As with inclusion, control types of interpersonal behaviour range on a continuum of controlling other people to not controlling anyone and being controlled by other people to not being controlled by other people. Three control types are identified and these are the abdicrat, the autocrat, and the democrat. The abdicrat control type is characterised by such behaviour as avoiding responsibility and power with a tendency to veer towards subordination. This type of person prefers others to take charge and consciously wanting to be relieved of any obligations because of their perceived lack of ability to carry out the responsibility. Autocrats on the other hand are the type of people who behave in a way to suggest total control and domination of other people with a strong desire to be at the top of the hierarchy. To put it simply these types of people are power seekers because they fear that people will not be influenced or controlled by them. Schutz (1966) sums the autocrat as 'no one thinks I can make decisions for myself, but I'll show them. I'm going to make all the decisions for everyone, always' (p. 29). The feeling that drives this type of person is one of distrust of others as well as perceived distrust from others. To put it simply, *I don't trust you but I know that you don't trust me.* As with the social type, democrats are those individuals who have successfully resolved their issues of control with others in childhood, thus power and control are not significant problems. These people are comfortable taking or not taking and giving or not giving orders. For Schutz (1966), the democrat 'unconsciously, he feels that he is a capable, responsible person and therefore that he does not need to shrink from responsibility or to try constantly to prove how competent he really is' (p. 30). Exercise 5 aims to situate the type of control within self.

EXERCISE 5

Reflect on your own interpersonal behaviour and how would you categorise your control type. For example, would you fit in abdicrat, democrat, or autocrat?

You may wish to reflect on some of the following: Do you for example try to

Dominate when you are with people or do you allow others to dominate?

Take charge when working in a group or do you allow other people to take charge?

Get others to do what you want or do you prefer others to tell you what to do?

Make decision or prefer others to make decisions for you?

Let other people influence what you do or do you prefer to influence what they do?

Would you describe yourself as follower or as a leader?

The interpersonal need for affection is seen as the need to establish and maintain satisfactory relationships with others concerning love and affection (Schutz, 1966). The two ends of the continuum of interpersonal need for affection are being comfortable with initiating close, personal relations with everyone to initiating close, personal relations with no one. Moreover, being comfortable with people when they initiate close, personal relations towards self to never originating close, personal relations towards self. The feeling aspect of interpersonal need for affection focuses on 'the need to establish and maintain a feeling of mutual affection with others' (Schutz, 1966, p. 20). Implicit with this feeling are being able to love other people to a reasonable degree and having others to love us to a reasonable degree. Linked to the notions of deficient, excessive, and ideal, the three types of affection are the underpersonal, the overpersonal, and the personal. Characteristically, those described as underpersonal tend to avoid close personal relationships with others. Relationship is always kept at a superficial level. These people are more comfortable when there is a reciprocal distancing of behaviour from other people. Schutz (1966) summarised the underpersonal as, 'I find the affection area very painful since I have been rejected; therefore I shall avoid close personal relations in the future' (p. 30). The overpersonal type of affection by contrast tries to become extremely close to other people. According to Schutz (1966), the type of people who fit this category tend to strive to be liked by others even to the extent of using subtle techniques such as manipulation, for example, 'to devour friends and subtly punish any attempts by them to establish other relationships, to be possessive' (Schutz, 1966, p. 31). Contrary to both the underpersonal and overpersonal, where unconsciously there is a strong need for affection, the personal affection type is attributed to those people who have successfully resolved their affectional relations with others in childhood and are thus comfortable with close emotional relations with others and this comfort translates to situations that require emotional distancing. It is important for personal people to be liked, however, it would not be the end of the world if this is not the case as they are quite clear in their minds that they are not unlovable people. Exercise 6 aims to situate the type of affection within self.

EXERCISE 6

Reflect on your own interpersonal behaviour, how would you categorise your affection type. For example, would you fit in underpersonal, personal, or overpersonal?

You may wish to reflect on some of the following: Do you, for example, try to

Be friendly with other people or are you cold and distant?

Have close relationships with others or do you prefer to your own company?

There is no scientific basis to Exercises 4–6, and these are only meant to help you to identify the type of inclusion you may fit in based on Schutz (1966) ideas. Whichever type of inclusion you consider yourself to be is only meant to be an awareness-raising exercise and not to be perceived as a negative or positive attribute. According to Schutz (1966), the relationship that we experienced in early childhood becomes our chosen model for our current interpersonal behaviour and will continue to be so throughout our life.[2]

Interpersonal styles

From what has been said so far it is clear that individuals have their own particular interpersonal needs that to a large extent dictate the way they behave when interacting with others. This phenomenon falls into the realm of interpersonal styles. According to Egan (1977) interpersonal style 'refers to the usual, the ordinary, the day-to-day ways in which you behave or act when you're with other people' (p. 14). Exercise 7 focuses on personal disclosure and requires self-reflection on past behaviour.

EXERCISE 7

How do you behave when you are in the following environment? (There is an assumption that our behaviour is different in various situations. This is a very general question; however, you may wish to work with one example.)
At home:
With friends:
At work:

The answers that you would have concluded from Exercise 7 would reveal your interpersonal style. Perhaps it would be true to say that there are qualitative differences in the way we behave at home, when we are with friends, or when we are at work. Home would probably be a much more conducive environment to disclose ourselves as we truly are. It could also be said that our behaviour with friends may not be as disclosing as it would be with our parents or intimate partners. At work, however, a great majority of what we do would be dictated by our professional code of conduct, hence may not be as revealing as when we are at home or with friends.

According to Egan (1977), the following types of questions would help in building your interpersonal style profile.[3]

1. How much of my life is my interpersonal life? Do I have a need to spend time with people or would I be more comfortable by myself?

2. What do I want and what do I need when I spend time with others? What do I see in them? Do they bring anything to the relationship?

3. Do I care about people in my life? How am I perceived in a relationship, selfless or self-centered?

4. How skilled am I at interpersonal communication? Have I the skills to show my understanding of others? Do I show them respect?

5. How close do I really want to be to other people? What does being close mean to me?

6. How do I deal with my emotions when I am in company of others? Am I perceived as a person with feelings or one who shows little emotion?

7. How do I behave in face of personal rejection? Am I bothered or not bothered?

8. Do I look for reciprocity in my relationships with others? Do I have ulterior motives in my behaviour or do I perceive others to have ulterior motives in their behaviour?

9. What is my relationship like at work or university? How do I feel in the presence of authority?

10. How do my interpersonal values influence my interaction with others? How honest and sincere am I in my relationships with others?

Interpersonal skills

Interpersonal skill or interpersonal competence could be described as the ability to comprehend the nature of social interactions, to be able to make an accurate judgement of the behaviour of others as well as being able to act in a way that enhances relationships. According to Trenholm and Jensen (2000), inter-personal competence has two levels. The first level relates to those observable behaviours and is called performative competence and the second level relates to cognitive activity that contributes to effective performance. Exercise 8 serves as a foundation for a discussion on some of the specific skills of interpersonal communication.

EXERCISE 8

To quote Trenholm and Jensen (2000), 'What does a person have to know or be able to do in order to communicate in a personally effective and socially appropriate manner?' (pp. 10–11).

Work out what you feel one needs to know and do in order to engage in interpersonal communication.

Your conclusion from Exercise 8 would lead to an insight into the notion of interpersonal skills. According to Hayes (1991), interpersonal skills are goal-directed behaviour that people engage in during an interpersonal interaction in order to reach a desired state of affairs. Here, however, the pressing question still remains *what is this goal-directed behaviour?* Implicit within the word skill is the notion of competence, and according to Adler and Rodman (2003), defining communication competence is not an easy task; however, if one achieves one's goals in such a way as to maintain or enhance the relationship in which it occurs, one would have achieved communication competence. For Trenholm and Jensen (2000), effective interpersonal communication is contingent upon five key skills and these are interpretive competence, goal competence, role competence, self-competence, and message competence. For the purpose of this discussion, henceforth these will be regarded as the core interpersonal skills.

Interpretive competence

Trenholm and Jensen (2000) describe this as a process of perceiving. Not too dissimilar to the concept of awareness that Egan (1977) argues under-pins every single interpersonal skill. Awareness or perception relates to a person's ability to make an accurate judgement of what is going on with another person as well as what is going on within oneself. Trenholm and Jensen (2000) explain the notion of interpretive competence as 'the ability to label, organize, and interpret the conditions surrounding an interaction; knowing how to size up people and situations' (p. 11). The implication is that it is only by sizing up our situation and the people we encounter with reasonable accuracy that enables us to demonstrate sensitivity towards others.

Most of the issues related to what goes on within oneself have already been addressed in Chapter 1 (Self-Awareness) and Chapter 7 (Intrapersonal Communication). Awareness of others requires the person to pay particular attention to people and their behaviour, thus enabling them to recognise any mismatch between verbal and non-verbal behaviour. For example, a patient may say, *I am all right* when in fact all the signs point to *I am anxious*. According to Egan (1977), 'learning how to pay closer attention to your-self, to others, and to the situations in which you find yourself relating to others is necessary if you're going to develop the kind of awareness that is the foundation of interpersonal skills' (p. 39). The skills of social and emotional intelligence (see Chapter 1) are significant in awareness of self and others. In answer to Trenholm and Jensen's (2000) question in relation to what does one have to know and do in order to communicate effectively with others, it could be said that perhaps none are more important than the skill of listening.

Listening skills

Hamachek (1991) states, 'probably no human behaviour is simultaneously as easy to do and yet as difficult to accomplish as listening, at least good listening' (p. 322). Perhaps Hayes (1991) is right when he says that people who cannot listen cannot relate. Imagine the following scenario. You have had a very hard morning at work and everything that could go wrong went wrong as a result you are feeling stressed. You decide to go and attempt to ventilate to one of your colleagues, Bob. You start to explain to Bob what your morning was like and well before you are able to finish Bob proceeds to tell you about his morning. What is interesting also is that Bob's morning appears to be much worse than yours. Although this scenario is purely hypothetical, personal encounters suggest that this would seem to be a common occurrence in our daily interactions with others. When this happens, one can't help but to wonder how much of what you have said has been listened to. In fact, perhaps we could safely conclude none at all because all Bob seemed to be interested in was to tell you about his morning. Exercise 9 may confirm the general lack of listening skills.

EXERCISE 9

The next time you encounter a colleague or a friend simply try and explain how much work you have to do and make a note of the reply you receive.

Our guess is that it will not be too dissimilar to the scenario presented above. Unfortunately, looking into the rationales for these types of behaviour is not within the scope of this chapter but suffice to stress that as a general rule people tend to function from an egocentric perspective as far as listening is concerned. According to Egan (1977), everyone has a craving to be understood and the only way we can understand them is by listening to what they have to say. 'Letting people know that I understand what they are saying to me is a kind of oil that lubricates the entire communication process' (Egan, 1977, p. 109). It could be argued that effective listening focuses on both feelings and content of a message. Moreover, it should not involve evaluation and judgement but simply an effort on the listener's part to try and understand what an individual is trying to communicate. According to Hamachek (1991), the purpose of listening is an effort on our part to inform others that we can accept and validate their feelings and ideas unconditionally. Total listening therefore can be defined as an active process that involves searching and capturing the true essence of what the speaker has said in relation to both content and feeling. Egan (1977) sees total listening as putting non-verbal behaviour, voice, and words together. Total listening involves what Hamachek (1991, p. 323) calls '*understanding responses*' which involve reflecting what the other person has said but using one's own words. Moreover, understanding responses are seen as an effective way to demonstrate total listening 'from the outside in, with no effort to prejudge the offering' (Hamachek, 1991, p. 323). Understanding responses are also seen as reflective responses that are defined as restating the feeling and content of the speaker's message in a way that demonstrates understanding and acceptance on the part of the listener. Another term that has similar meaning to reflective or understanding responses is empathic listening, which suggests listening in order to understand the other person's point of view. According to Trenholm and Jensen (2000), empathic listening is the one type of listening that closely relates to improving interpersonal communication and more so when emotions are involved. To this end Trenholm and Jensen (2000) suggest the following four guiding principles.

1. Respect the other person's point of view.

2. Make sure we fully understand what has been said before responding.

3. Check our understanding by paraphrasing.

4. Paraphrasing would need to include relational as well as content message.

Content message can be described as what is actually being said, similar to a verbatim transcript of what one hears. Relational messages on the other hand serve to situate content messages in context. As Trenholm and Jensen (2000) state, 'they let us know whether a statement is a put-down, a sincere overture of friendship, a sarcastic retort, or a joke' (p. 114). For example, someone's content message may be *I would like to have a chat with you but I can see you are busy so I shall come back another time. Don't worry it can wait*, but then the person leaves with tears in his or her eyes. Here, the content message is saying one thing and the relational message is saying another. According to Watzlawick, Bavelas, and Jackson (1967), content messages are usually expressed in verbal forms whereas relational messages are sent non-verbally and often unconsciously. Verbal and non-verbal communication are discussed later in this chapter.

Goal competence

The notion of goal competence implies one's ability to set a goal and to anticipate its possible outcome as well as choosing an effective course of action (Trenholm & Jensen, 2000). This implies that people would need to establish the why of their communication and work out a strategy for achieving their identified goal. For example, if the objective of communication is to influence another person into doing something then one would need to have a plan of action as to what to do or say in order to reach that end. According to Trenholm and Jensen (2000), the starting point of influencing another person rests with a knowledge of that person's needs, for example, the need for rewards, the need for stability and consistency, and the need for self-respect.

The need for rewards

It is clear that people, in general, tend to behave according to what Thorndike's (1911) describes as the law of effect. The implication is that we are most likely to repeat a behaviour if the outcome is positive than if the outcome is negative. This principle is discussed fully in Chapter 4 as underpinning the notion of operant conditioning that explains some of the interpersonal behaviour such as entering into or dissolving a relationship. Moreover, classical conditioning, social learning (see Chapter 4 for explanation of both these concepts), and social exchange theory also contribute to an understanding of interpersonal processes. According to Emerson (1972) the development of social exchange theory is credited to four theorists, George Homans (1961), John Thibaut and Harrold Kelly (1959), and Peter Blau (1964) based on the notion that our behaviour is contingent on rewarding reactions from others or as Trenholm and Jensen (2000) put it 'if given a choice between two relationships, we will choose the more rewarding one' (p. 231). However, Emerson (1972), warns that the exchange theory should not be taken as a theory per se. It should instead be seen as a frame of reference that takes the movement of valued things through social process as its focus. The implication is that generally speaking people will always do something provided their behaviour is reinforced. Reinforcement is taken to mean positively rewarded.

The need for stability and consistency

According to Heider (1958), people have a need for maintaining harmony among such things as perceptions, beliefs, and attitudes. For example, if we like someone and that someone shares similar attitudes to ourselves then we are said to be in balance that is there exists a consistency between liking someone and his or her attitude (consistency theory was discussed in Chapter 7). However, a state of imbalance is created when we like someone only to discover that he or she holds opposite attitudes to ourselves. A similar state of imbalance is present when we dislike someone who holds similar attitudes to ourselves. In both these instances we are faced with inconsistencies that we dislike and feel uncomfortable (see cognitive dissonance theory in Chapter 7).

The need for self-respect

Self-respect is inextricably linked with self-concept and in particular with the self-esteem component (self-esteem is briefly discussed in Chapter 1 and the notion of respect forms part of the discussion in Chapter 9). As with self-acceptance, if individuals can't respect themselves for who they are, then it becomes problematic for them to respect others. This sentiment is captured by Hamachek (1991) who states, 'respect for one's own integrity and uniqueness, love and understanding of one's own self, cannot be separated from respect and love and understanding for another individual' (p. 328). It could be said that if we can come to appreciate ourselves for whom we are, including our inherent worth without imposing any self-deprecation, then our journey to self-respect has already begun. However, lack of self-respect leads to low self-esteem and in turn to negative self-concept.

Role competence

Roles are important in life because they help to clarify people's expectation of behaviour in society. For example, our expectation of health care professionals is that they would behave as therapeutic agents. To this end, therefore, it could be said that roles define patterns of behaviour expected of its members (Adler & Rodman, 2003). Role is also seen to be closely linked to the concept of institution. For example, given that hospital is an institution it has clearly defined roles for its employees. The notion of role competence therefore rests with each employee's ability to take on his or her social or professional role and to know what is appropriate behaviour for that given role (Trenholm & Jensen, 2000). Every discipline has its own professional body to define its code of conduct, for example doctors have the General Medical Council, nurses and midwives have The Nursing and Midwifery Council, and the same would apply for other disciplines such as audiology, radiology, and so on. As health care professionals, therefore, we would each need to ask ourselves *what do I need to know in order to be able to do my job effectively?* From a health care perspective, Egan (1977) posits that communication know-how is a requisite for every role and this suggests one's ability to translate awareness of self and of others as well as its underpinning knowledge to actual interactions. Moreover, this would need to include knowledge of the content of what is being communicated. For example, a doctor must be competent in medical knowledge, a nurse must be competent in nursing knowledge, a midwife must be competent in knowledge of midwifery, an audiologist must be competent in knowledge of audiology, and so on and so forth. Egan (1977) states that one's accurate perception is useless 'if they remain locked up inside you because you don't know how to express them' (p. 39). Accurate perception of others and the situation in which they find themselves could be linked with the notion of empathic understanding (see Chapter 1) as a key skill for health care professionals that Berlo (1960) sums up as 'the ability to project ourselves into other people's personalities' (p. 119). There are at least two theories of empathy, the inference theory and the role taking theory.

The principal assumptions of the inference theory of empathy are as follows.

- People have first evidence of their own internal states. They can only have second-hand evidence of other people's internal states. This implies that people's first-hand knowledge is of themselves and any other knowledge comes second.

- Other people express a given internal state by performing the same behaviour that you perform to express the same state. This, according to Berlo (1960), seems to be implying that everyone expresses the same meaning by the same behaviour and vice versa. To assume that we all attach the same meaning to the same set of behaviour is misleading in that we fail to take into account this *particular kind of person*. In order to understand the notion of empathy, we need to reject this idea that, people's first-hand knowledge is always used principally because we are unique and as such it does not necessarily follow that what we come to know about ourselves in a given situation can equate to what others are experiencing in a similar situation.

- People cannot understand internal states in other people that they themselves have not experienced. It would be fair to say that people have greater understanding of the things that they have experienced. However, it would also be true to say that people do understand, if not wholly then partly, what other people are experiencing at a given point in their lives. For example, we don't all have to win the lottery to know how good it must feel to have won. Moreover, we don't have to experience loss to understand what it must feel like to lose someone we are close to. As Berlo (1960) states, 'experience increases our understanding, but it does not seem to be essential to understanding' (p. 124).

The role-taking theory of empathy contends that the concept of self does not precede communication. It is instead developed through communication. For example, the infants play other people's roles without interpretation such as when they imitate behaviour of others. Gradually, the infant progresses to role-playing with understanding and eventually moves on to 'put himself in other people's shoes symbolically, rather than physically' (Berlo, 1960, p. 126).

Self-competence

This can be described as one's ability to choose and portray a desired self-image. According to Trenholm and Jensen (2000), one of the most important aspects of growing up is developing a sense of individuality and personal communication style, central to which is the development of a healthy self-concept (see Chapter 1). The notion of self-efficacy would also help to clarify self-competence.

It could be argued that competencies influence expectancies and vice versa. For example, if I believe that I am competent the likelihood is that I will try difficult tasks. Bandura (1982) calls this phenomenon self-efficacy expectation. 'People tend to avoid situations they believe exceed their coping capabilities, but they undertake and perform assuredly activities they judge themselves capable of managing' (Bandura, Reese, & Adams, 1982, p. 5). It could also be argued that self-efficacy expectation leads to persistent and assertive behaviour in that people will try harder and with much more conviction. As Bandura, Reese, and Adams (1982) explain, self-judged efficacy determines the amount of effort people will exert and 'how long they will persist in the face of obstacles or aversive experiences' (p. 5). The notion of assertiveness suggests acting in one's best interest without undue anxiety and to express one's honest feeling comfortably or to exercise one's rights without denying the rights of others (Alberti & Emmons, 1970). Behaviour can be observed on a continuum that starts from a non-assertive position (submissive) through to aggressive and the halfway point being assertive. According to Egan (1977), whenever we allow other people to walk all over us without so much as an attempt to protect our rights we assume the submissive position. By contrast, when we walk all over others in order to satisfy our needs we take on an aggressive position. Raw assertiveness without awareness and without communication know-how turns a person into a potentially destructive communicator (Egan, 1977).

Message competence

The ability to speak a language that other people can understand and respond to falls into the realm of message competence, principally defined as verbal and non-verbal skills. Verbal skill can be described as people's ability to use speech to express meaning effectively. Similarly, non-verbal skill relates to people's ability to use non-speech or non-words. According to Trenholm and Jensen (2000), verbal and non-verbal codes combine to convey content meaning that consists of both the ideas and the feeling of the speaker (for example, what is being said) and relational meaning that is more contextual in that it defines the relationship with the speaker (as in how it is being said).

Verbal and non-verbal communication

Verbal forms of communication have speech and language as their foundations. Language is the topic of Chapter 6. The focus here is on non-verbal communication and competence. Initially however, we need to explore the fundamental difference between verbal and non-verbal channels that according to Danziger (1976) function on two entirely different coding principles. For example, verbal messages use digital coding while non-verbal messages are based on analogic codes. Digital coding is seen as arbitrary because they hold no resemblance with the item they represent. Digital codes are merely symbols used to represent something but cannot be seen as the thing itself. For example, the combination of the digits b-o-o-k is only meant to represent book but in themselves they do not resemble a real book. As Trenholm and Jensen (2000) state, 'symbols are conventional, based on social agreement. We could easily change the meaning attached to the words in our language – if everyone within our language community agreed' (p. 86). This was the case with the word marathon, a race run over a distance of 46 kilometres. However, when a chocolate bar was named Marathon (now known as Snickers) its meaning changes from a race to a chocolate. Analogic upon which non-verbal is based on the other hand does resemble the thing that it represents. For example, a painful expression on someone's face represents the felt emotion of pain. Verbally, the individual may say *I am fine* but visually one can read *I am in pain*. According to Egan (1977), if our facial expression gives a different message from the words we speak, most people will believe what they see on our faces. This implies that non-verbal communication is considered to be much more powerful than verbal communication. We may be good at bending the truth with the words that we use; however, we will find it difficult, if not impossible, to do the same with some of our non-verbal behaviour principally because these are not always conscious and as such have a tendency to escape our effort to deceive. This phenomenon is commonly referred to as non-verbal leakage (Ekman & Friesen, 1969). A further type of communication relates to the non-linguistic aspects of speech commonly referred to as paralanguage where the same word may be said in several aspects of voice quality thus conveying different meanings (Argyle, 1972). Paralanguage among other factors involves loudness, pitch, and speed such as pauses between words or sentences.

There are two schools of thought into what constitute non-verbal communication. The first is broader and based on the premise that any behaviour that a receiver perceives is communication, the inclusion of unintentional behaviour is seen by some theorists as non-verbal communication. For example, a frown may be unintentional nevertheless it conveys a sense of disapproval or displeasure, hence the communication of a message. The second is narrower and argues that communication per se only relates to intentional behaviour therefore a frown may not be seen as non-verbal communication. However, Burgoon (1985) offers a more comprehensive explanation that situate both intentional and unintentional behaviour in the context of non-verbal communication, for example,

> what qualifies as communication are those behavior that form a socially shared coding system; that is, they are behaviors that are typically sent with intent, used with regularity among members of a social community, are typically interpreted as intentional, and have consensually recognizable interpretations . . . . The key word is 'typically.' If a behavior is usually encoded deliberately and is usually interpreted as meaningful by receivers or observers, it does not matter if, on a given occasion, it is performed unconsciously or unintentionally; it still qualifies as a message.
>
> (Knapp & Miller, 1985, p. 348)

This position is favoured in any discussion relating to the theme of non-verbal communication throughout this book.

Functions of non-verbal communication

According to Burgoon (1985), non-verbal behaviour operates as an integrated and coordinated way in order to achieve their particular social functions that include expressing meaning, formation and management of impression, and structuring and regulating the flow of interaction.

Non-verbal communication as an expression of meaning

This is especially the case in the domains of emotion and attitude. For example, it would not be difficult to recognise a face that expresses anger or one that expresses disgust. In fact, Aaronson, Wilson, and Akert (1997), describe the face as the crown jewel of non-verbal communication. Moreover, there is an element of universality about facial expression in that there are at least six major emotions that are said to be cross-cultural and these are happiness, sadness, fear, anger, disgust, and surprise (Ekman, Friesen, & Ellsworth, 1982). Similarly, people's facial expression will also indicate their likes or dislikes of an object. For example, a smile may reveal approval, whereas a stern face may suggest otherwise.

Non-verbal communication as formation and management of impression

The notion of impression formation was introduced in Chapter 7. A brief account is given here in relation to how non-verbal behaviour can help to form and manage impression. According to Burgoon (1985), when we meet other people for the first time we engage in a reciprocal process of impression formation in relation to age, gender, socio-economic-status, ethnicity, and geographical residence. However, we tend to pay more attention to non-verbal cues than speech because as Burgoon states, 'initial verbal exchanges are so often constrained by conventions' (Knapp & Miller, 1985, p. 372). This would seem to suggest that we are verbally very guarded in what we say and how much we say about ourselves. Moreover, it is much more difficult to manipulate non-verbal cues, such as the way we look (as in body type), our facial attractiveness, our hairstyle, the way we dress, and even our accent. Interestingly, it is possible to manage the impression that we would like other people to have of us. Jones and Pittman (1982) identified five key areas that people usually engage in when trying to manage the impression they make on others. These are as follows.

■ *Self-promotion* indicates people's primary goal would be to portray themselves as competent, for example they may verbalise their achievements as well as what they are capable of. Non-verbally, these could be in the form of displaying their certificates, awards, or posters in full view for everyone to see. Such behaviour, for example, being more animated, smiles more, and a relaxed posture are said to display positive images of self. This is validated by Howard and Ferris (1996), who reported that applicants who use positive non-verbals such as smiling, head nodding, and direct eye gaze are seen as more competent than those who use negative non-verbals such as avoiding eye contact.

■ *Ingratiation* suggests that people would try to get into other people's good books by doing them favours or using flattery to be perceived in a positive light. Non-verbally, they would give frequent eye gaze to demonstrate great interest in what the other person is doing or saying. Similarly, if we were to do something for you that you yourself cannot do chances are you will like us more. We are, as Cialdini (1993) calls it, 'phenomenal suckers for flattery' (p. 175).

- *Examplification* means people would put themselves out in order to give the message that they are dedicated to what they do. Non-verbally this could be seen in such behaviour as working overtime without any financial reward or as Rosenfeld, Giacalone, and Riordan (2002) explain 'the co-worker who takes work home every day, and the colleague who never takes a vacation' (p. 69).

- *Intimidation* implies that people would let others know that they are the boss and that they have the potential to punish if the need arises. Non-verbally, intimidators can be unpredictable. Moreover, the use of silent stares is often used as a tactic to intimidate. Other non-verbal behaviour would include looking threatening, hard face, and with no smiles.

- *Supplication* suggests people would give the message that they have weaknesses and that they need others. For example, people would exploit their own weaknesses to influence others. Non-verbally this could be displayed in any behaviour that carries the following sentiment, *if I play the victim, this forces you to be my rescuer.* Moreover, there are always people out there who will willingly help someone who needs it. Exercise 10 could prove interesting.

EXERCISE 10

Reflect on your entourage and identify one of the following types of individual:

Self-promoter
Ingratiator
Examplificator
Intimidator
Supplicator.

Non-verbal communication as structuring and regulating the flow of interaction

According to Burgoon (1985), structuring and regulating the flow of interaction can be seen in defining situation and defining role relationships. Architectural features may indicate the nature of the interaction, for example whether this is formal or informal. Moreover, physical attractiveness may dictate whether contact will be made or not. According to Trenholm and Jensen (2000), non-verbal communication is principally responsible for the smoothness of turn taking when two people are in conversation.

Types of non-verbal communication

There are numerous types of non-verbal communication and these include proxemics, posture and gesture, touch, facial expression, eye gaze, and appearance (including physical attractiveness and clothing). Moreover, all are revealing in the way they convey information and their importance cannot be underestimated. In-depth discussion on all non-verbal behaviour is beyond the scope of this chapter. The following paragraphs address the notions of proxemics and posture, concluding with a brief explanation on gesture.

Proxemics (distance)

Individuals have always made clear their need for space in the way they position themselves in relation to others. The systematic study of these spatial features of social presentation is what Hall (1959) calls proxemics and is sometimes referred to as interpersonal distance. For example, during an interaction with another person, both individuals would attempt to maintain a certain distance that they are comfortable with. It is argued that interpersonal distance is individually as well as culturally defined. For example, what suits one individual may not necessarily suit another. Exercise 11 offers some insight into the notion of interpersonal distance.

EXERCISE 11

Perhaps you could enlist the help of one of your colleagues. Ask your colleague to stand approximately six or seven feet away from you. Then gradually move towards your colleague to the first point where you (or your colleague) start to feel uncomfortable. Make an approximate guess of the distance.

According to Danziger (1976), the usual distance in ordinary conversation is four to five feet and variations of more than some inches either way lead to feelings of discomfort. However, violation of what Danziger (1976, p. 59) calls 'the unwritten rules of interpersonal distance' never goes unnoticed, for example, no sooner someone encroaches upon our personal space we retreat in an attempt to maintain this personal distance. Moreover, the narrower the interpersonal distance the higher the degree of intimacy. Numerous factors come into play in defining one's personal boundary and these include the nature of relationship with the other person, the physical surroundings, and culture. According to Argyle (1972), physical proximity is one of the cues for intimacy of both a sexual nature and between friends. Close proximity to the point of body contact, as is often the case in a lift or crowded places seems to be a 'permissible' violation of personal space principally because it has 'no affiliative significance' (Argyle, 1972, p. 37). The implication is that body contact in this context amounts to nothing, interestingly, however, we tend to protect ourselves in other ways as in

Table 8.1 The dynamism of space based on the idea of Hall (1966)

Zone		Distance	Characteristics
Intimate	Close	Full body contact	As in love making, hugging, and reserved for people whom we are emotionally close to. There are exceptions, for example, the 'unwritten rule' that allows health care professionals permission to enter this intimate zone.
	Far	6–8 inches	
Personal	Close	1½–2½ Feet	This space can be seen as 'a small protective sphere or bubble that an organism maintains between itself and others' (Hall, 1966, p. 112). However, this distance is sufficiently close to reach out to someone and far enough to keep people at arm's length should they choose to do so. Far phase is seen as the limit of physical domination. Topics of mutual interest can be discussed. Each other's detail features are clearly visible. Similarly, body and breath odour can be detected.
	Far	2½–4 feet	
Social	Close	4–7 feet	Intimate visual detail is not easily perceived. Physical contact is not possible except with great effort. Generally, one does not have to raise voice at the close phase but may have to do so at the far phase. Impersonal business takes place at the close phase. Social distance is culturally defined at any phase. The far phase offers individuals opportunity to engage or disengage in conversation at will.
	Far	7–12 feet	
Public	Close	12–25 feet	Individuals are far enough to take flight if they so wish. Voice would need to be louder than normal. Visual details are lost in the far phase. More effort is needed to convey the message of communication.
	Far	25 feet or more	

The hidden dimension: Man's use of space in public and private. London, Sydney, and Toronto: The Bodley Head.

avoiding conversation as well as avoiding eye contact (Table 8.1). Hall (1966) highlights four distances that are used in North American culture and each of these distances has a close and far phase as seen in Table 8.1.

General observation suggests that when people's space is invaded they are most likely to show signs of discomfort and are inclined to take evasive or protective action as you may have concluded from Exercise 11. However, evasive action may not be possible for some patients especially those who are deemed to be a danger to themselves and placed under close observation. Research suggest that patients feel as if the person observing them is right in their face (Cardell & Pitula, 1999). Exercise 12 offers an opportunity to imagine the effect of invasion of your personal space.

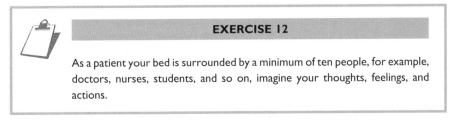

EXERCISE 12

As a patient your bed is surrounded by a minimum of ten people, for example, doctors, nurses, students, and so on, imagine your thoughts, feelings, and actions.

From Exercise 12, the feeling of being crowded in is most likely to be experienced. Crowding can be described as the psychological state of discomfort and stress associated with the spatial aspects of the environment (Sears, Peplau, & Freedman, 1988).

Posture (bodily posture)

Posture is often seen as body language that reveals information within the context of a given situation. The way individuals sit, walk, and generally conduct themselves all have their own stories to tell. For example, it would not be difficult to tell when someone is uncomfortable, anxious, in pain, or in a rush. The information that body posture conveys can compliment or contradict verbal messages. While verbal language may be manipulated to distort the truth, body language *tells it as it is*. You may find Exercise 13 interesting.

EXERCISE 13

Have a look at Figure 8.1 and identify what messages you feel these convey.

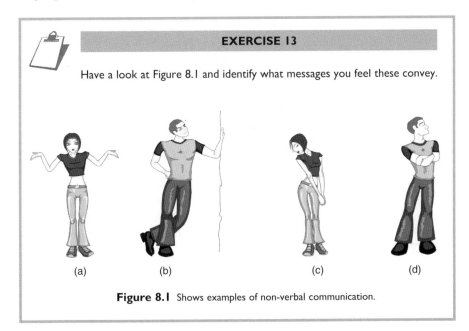

(a)   (b)   (c)   (d)

Figure 8.1 Shows examples of non-verbal communication.

According to Mehrabian (1972), body language gives an idea of the immediacy that exists between two individuals demonstrating the physical closeness that they allow with others and this includes touching, distance, forward lean towards the other person, eye contact, and body orientation. The implication is that 'increasing immediacy corresponds to greater degree of touching, forward lean, eye contact and directness of body orientation, and smaller distances' (Mehrabian, 1972, pp. 25–26). Other functions include agreement or disagreement and power or authority. Reflecting on Exercise 13 and based on the work of Argyle (1972) Figure 8.1a represents someone who is disinterested, doubtful, and questioning. People also tend to adopt this type of position when there are describing an event. Figure 8.1b on the other hand may represent someone who is self-satisfied or impatient. People who are angry may also exhibit this posture. Figure 8.1c is the classic posture for someone who is shy, self-conscious, ashamed, modest, or sad. Figure 8.1d represents someone who is surprised, dominating, or suspicious.

While posture relates to the position of the whole body, gesture applies to only part (or parts) of the body. Lamb and Watson (1979) describe posture and gesture in terms of *having* and *making*, respectively, for example one can have a posture but would need to make a gesture. Gestures can be described as movements of hands, feet, or other parts of the body. Some are intended to communicate definite messages such as raising a clenched fist (aggression) or waving an arm (saying goodbye). Others are seen as involuntary social cues that may or may not be accurately be interpreted by others (Argyle, 1972).

Summary

The very essence of communication rests with the notion that messages are sent and received in the manner that they are intended. Communication as emphasised in this chapter is interpersonal suggesting an element of closeness in the way individuals interact with one another. Person is not seen just as person but instead as someone with special characteristics that differentiate him or her from others. Therefore the goal of interpersonal communication is to recognise and validate an individual's unique sense of being. Three interpersonal needs are highlighted as inclusion, control, and affection and these tend to dictate the way people interact with one another. Effective interpersonal communication has its foundation in the core skills of interpretive, goal, role, self, and message competences translated through verbal, non-verbal, and paralanguages.

References

Aaronson, E., Wilson, T. D., and Akert, R. M. (1997). *Social Psychology*. New York: Longman.

Adler, R. B. and Rodman, G. (2003). *Understanding Human Communication*. New York and Oxford: Oxford University Press.

Alberti, R. E. and Emmons, M. L. (1970). *Your Perfect Right: A Guide to Assertive Behaviour*. San Luis, Obsipo: Impact.

Argyle, M. (1972). *The Psychology of Interpersonal Behaviour*. London, Reading, and Fakenham: Penguin Books.

Bandura, A. (1982). Self-efficacy mechanism in human agency. *American Psychologist*, 37, 122–147.

Bandura, A., Reese, L., and Adams, N. E. (1982). Microanalysis of action and fear arousal as a function of different levels of perceived self-efficacy. *Journal of Personality and Social Psychology*, 43, 5–21.

Berenson, F. M. (1981). *Understanding Persons: Personal and Impersonal Relations.* Brighton: Harvester.

Berlo, D. K. (1960). *The Process of Communication: An Introduction to Theory and Practice.* New York: Holt, Rinehart, and Winston.

Blau, P. (1964). *Exchange and Power in Social Life.* New York and London: Wiley.

Bochner, A. P. (1985). Perspectives on inquiry: representation, conversation, and reflection. In M. L. Knapp and G. R. Miller (eds.), *Handbook of Interpersonal Communication* (pp. 27–58). Beverly Hills, London, and New Delhi: Sage Publications.

Burgoon, J. K. (1985). Nonverbal signals. In M. L. Knapp and G. R. Miller (eds.), *Handbook of Interpersonal Communication* (pp. 344–390). Beverly Hills, London, and New Delhi: Sage Publications.

Cardell, R. and Pitula, C. R. (1999). Suicidal Inpatients' perceptions of therapeutic and nontherapeutic aspects of constant observation. *Psychiatric Services*, 50(8), 1066–1070.

Cialdini, R. B. (1993). *Influence: The Psychology of Persuasion.* New York: William Morrow and Company, Inc.

Danziger, K. (1976). *Interpersonal Communication.* New York, Toronto, Oxford, Sydney, Paris, and Braunschweig: Pergamon Press Inc.

Duck, S. (1999). *Relating to Others.* Buckingham and Philadelphia: Open University Press.

Egan, G. (1977). *You & Me: The Skills of Communicating and Relating to Others.* Monterey: Brooks/Cole Publishing Company.

Ekman, P. and Friesen, W. V. (1969). Non-verbal leakage and clues to deception. *Psychiatry*, 32, 88–105.

Ekman, P., Friesen, W. V., and Ellsworth, P. (1982). What are the similarities and differences in facial behaviour across cultures? In P. Ekman (ed.), *Emotions in Human Face* (pp. 128–143). Cambridge, England: Cambridge University.

Emerson, R. M. (1972). Exchange theory. Part 1: a psychological basis for social exchange and exchange theory. In J. Berger, M. Zelditch, and B. Anderson (eds.), *Sociological Theories in Progress* (Vol. 2, pp. 38–57). Boston: Houghton-Mifflin and Co.

Hall, E. T. (1959). The Silent Language. Garden City: Doubleday.

Hall, E. T. (1966). *The Hidden Dimension* (pp. 133–134). Garden City: Doubleday.

Hamachek, D. (1991). *Encounters with Self.* Fort Worth, New York, London, Sydney, and Tokyo: Harcourt Brace Jovanovich College Publishers.

Hayes, J. (1991). *Interpersonal Skills: Goal Directed Behaviour at Work.* London: Harper Collins Academics.

Heider, F. (1958). *The Psychology of Interpersonal Relations.* New York: John Wiley and Sons, Inc.

Homans, G. C. (1961). *Social Behaviour: Its Elementary Forms.* London: Routledge and Kegan Paul.

Howard, J. L. and Ferris, G. R. (1996). The employment interview context: social and situational influences on interviewer decisions. *Journal of Applied Social Psychology*, 26, 112–136.

Jones, E. E. and Pittman, T. S. (1982). Toward a general theory of strategic self-presentation. In J. Suls (ed.), *Psychological Perspectives on the Self* (pp. 231–261). Hillsdale: Lawrence Erlbaum.

Knapp, M. L. and Miller, G. R. (ed.) (1985). *Handbook of Interpersonal Communication.* Beverly Hills, London, and New Delhi: Sage Publications.

Lamb, W. and Watson, E. (1979). *Body Code: the Meaning in Movement.* London, Boston, and Henley: Routledge and Kegan Paul.

Maslow, A. H. (1968). *Towards a Psychology or Being.* New York: Van Nostrand.

Maslow, A. H. (1999). *Toward a Psychology of Being* (3rd edition). New York, Chichester, Weinheim, Brisban, Singapore, and Toronto: John Wiley and Sons, Inc.

Mehrabian, A. (1972). *Nonverbal Communication.* Chicago and New York: Aldine Atherton, Inc.

Murira, N., Lutzen, K., Lindmark, G., and Christensson, K. (2003). Communication pattern between health care providers and their clients at an antenatal clinic in Zimbabwe. *Health Care for Women International*, 24, 83–92.

Rosenfeld, P., Giacalone, R. A., and Riordan, C. A. (2002). Impression management: building and enhancing reputations at work. Australia, United Kingdom, and United States: Thomson Learning.

Schutz, W. C. (1966). Chapter 5. In *The Interpersonal Underworld*. Palo Alto: Science & Behaviour Books, Inc.

Sears, O. D., Peplau, A., and Freedman, J. (1988). *Social Psychology*. Englewood Cliffs: Prentice Hall.

Thibaut, J. W. and Kelly, H. (1959). *The Social Psychology of Groups*. New York, London, and Sydney: John Wiley and Sons.

Thorndike, E. L. (1911). *Animal Intelligent: Experimental Studies*. New York: Macmillan Press.

Trenholm, S. and Jensen, A. (2000). *Interpersonal Communication*. Belmont: Wadsworth.

Watzlawick, P., Bavelas, J. B., and Jackson, D. D. (1967). *Pragmatics of Human Communication*. New York: Norton.

Engagement and Developing Relationships

Dev M. Rungapadiachy

After reading this chapter you should be able to

■ Discuss the notion of relationship building in a collaborative partnership.

■ Translate your theoretical understanding of the process of engagement and relationship building to your clinical practice.

Introduction

There is no doubt that the process of engagement rests with effective communication. This means that both health care professionals and patients would need to speak the same language (Chapter 6). Health care professionals would need to recognise and respect patient's values (Chapter 7) and demonstrate the skills of interpersonal communication (Chapter 8). Chapter 9 attempts to situate the notion of engagement within the concept of care through a structured approach based on the notion of therapeutic relationship and partners in care.

From health to ill health: Patient experience

What does it mean to be healthy? This should not be a difficult question to answer because most of us are aware that to feel healthy is to feel reasonably unhindered. For example, a healthy status frees an individual to do almost anything he or she chooses. For Peplau (1988), health is 'a symbol that implies a forward movement of personality and other on-going processes in a direction of creative, constructive, productive personal and community living' (p. 12). This would seem to fit with the idea that a healthy person is free and autonomous (presented in Part II). The next question, however, might not be that straight forward as may be the case with Exercise 1.

EXERCISE I

What does it mean for you to suffer ill health?

It could be argued that only those who suffer or who have suffered ill health can be in a position to answer this question with reasonable accuracy and even then it is likely that answers will vary. For example, some may see ill health as an inconvenience (*as in I have so much to do and being ill is getting in the way*) or lack of security (*will my illness jeopardise my job prospect?*) while others, for example, doctors see it as 'difficult', 'embarrassing', and even 'shocking', with the degree of discomfort likely to be related to the uncertainty inherent in illness itself, the gravity of the condition and the stigmatising power of certain disorders (McKevitt & Morgan, 1997, p. 648). It would not be an exaggeration to say that illness brings with it a sense of loss, emotional arousal of anger, and feeling of disempowerment. These factors are compounded by the adoption of the patient or 'sick role' as coined by Parsons (1951). Parsons defines sickness as a threat to the sense of interpersonal responsibility that each individual holds. Being sick provides individuals with a legitimate reason (validated by a sick note from the doctor) for withdrawing from their role obligations. 'For this reason it requires systematic regulation to prevent it being used as an excuse for getting out of customary duties' (Hart, 1985, p. 97). Not surprising therefore that the patient role carries its own stigma regardless of the illness one happens to suffer from. However, this stigma can be more pronounced in certain illness, for example sexually transmitted diseases, hepatitis B, epilepsy, mental illness, etc. Stigma aside, the mere entry to any health care environment can itself be problematic in that it symbolises disempowerment that increases further a patient's vulnerability to stress. The experience of vulnerability is believed to create stress and anxiety that affect physiological, psychological, and social functioning. Moreover, individuals are vulnerable at different times in their lives, and illness would be such a time. As argued in Chapter 2, some people are likely to be more affected than others. Vulnerability, as previously discussed, includes numerous factors and one such factor is the environment. Patients will derive some sense of comfort from a supportive environment and possibly an increase level of discomfort from one that is perceived as hostile as exemplified by Russell (1999) who found her patients' experience of treatment in intensive care units to include encountering staff who seemed to adopt the *could not be bothered to talk attitude*. Other patients reported being afraid, in pain, and suffer discomfort as a result of the treatment. Still others felt alone without their loved ones. It could be argued that the key to good care and treatment is to have some grasp of what patients may be experiencing during the course of their illness. The word empathy captures this sentiment that is clearly obvious in the following extract from Griffiths's (2007) 'Uncomfortable experiences'.

I understand the need for experience. As in many walks of life often experience is the only way of learning. One aspect of being a medical student, however, I find awkward at best. I am not lambasting the ruthless consultants, because I have found them to be a far throw from their stereotype. They generally accept the limitations of my knowledge – that although I know my 'arse from my elbow' I do not know my maximus from my minimus, my pneumonia from my pneumothorax, and so on. I enjoy the experience gained from speaking to them and the demonstrations they do on patients. My unease comes from the medical student–patient relationship, a situation that you can only describe as tricky. It is often an awkward concoction of taboos, inappropriate questions, and misguided palpitations. Unlike a doctor, I offer no service to the patient. Patients are in fact doing me a service by giving consent for me to take a history or to do an examination. As a result I feel obliged to cause patients as little trouble as possible. This contradicts the objective of the exercise because to reach a diagnosis certain questions need to be asked and examinations done. I am meant to be gaining the experience of a doctor doing the same task. Doctors have the confidence of their profession, and the patient depends on them to ask any question and do any examination that is appropriate. I know that I should ask about a patient's smoking in relation to their cough, wheeze, and colourful sputum. If left to my own devices, however, without the pressure of a doctor evaluating my performance, I would much prefer to assume the habits of a patient with chronic obstructive pulmonary disease, rather than making a patient suffer the indignity of admitting their weaknesses to a fresh faced, white coated student.

When, or indeed if, I am a doctor, this situation will no longer occur because my actions will have more purpose. This reaction is not because of a lack of confidence on my part. Hours of 'personal development' have helped me to 'get in touch with myself' and overcome any problems I may have had with communication. In fact, I have become acutely aware of a sense of discomfort on the part of the patient. This is particularly pertinent in very ill patients who are at their most vulnerable and who already have their inadequacies and disabilities on display. I often wonder why patients volunteer to participate in such a process. For the more alert patients, and patients in less discomfort, I think it acts as a welcome distraction from the day's mundane blend of crosswords, catheters, and ciprofloxacin. These patients are usually more approachable and less embarrassed. Some also appreciate the need for medical students to gain experience and willingly do their bit for the medical profession. Another group doesn't have the ability to say no. Whichever way you take that, it does not bode well for a comfortable patient. A good example is that of an elderly foreign woman, who had, among many other problems, a 'fantastic' murmur. I can confidently say even with my limited medical knowledge that she was terminally ill. But the news of her defect had travelled throughout the hospital, and by the time I arrived in my group of eight, a queue had already formed. We bided our time with an elderly man blessed with a boring, normal heart before it was finally our turn. The doctor said, 'Just let me know if you have had enough', and he lifted up her top to expose her aged breast, hoisted it up, and located the murmur. As I approached I felt like a juror casting my vote for the death penalty while questioning the verdict. I politely warmed my stethoscope and placed it on her chest with a smile and muttered words of thanks.

She looked straight ahead with a look of anguish, boredom, and fear. As I scuttled back to the safety of the group it struck me that a diagnosis was being made and a worsening prognosis every time a diaphragm was placed on her chest. Imagine lying in hospital and 30 people in white coats approach you, listen to your heart, and then nod as they confirm the severity of your problem. With every student you become more abnormal, more exposed, and less treatable.

Capacity, a requisite for informed consent, should be applied more stringently when finding patients for students. It should also accommodate the idea that a patient may be afraid or reluctant to say no to a doctor. Not all patients who present to us are entirely willing or suitable for us to examine. You could say that the job means having to meet all kinds of people and that therefore it is a valuable exercise in gaining experience. But it is not my discomfort that concerns me, it is that of the patient.

(Griffiths, 2007, p. 35) Reproduced with permission from
the BMJ Publishing Group.[1]

Exercise 2 offers an opportunity to further analyse what it may feel like to *be a patient*.

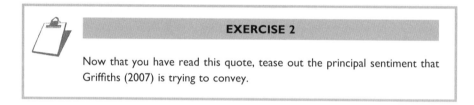

EXERCISE 2

Now that you have read this quote, tease out the principal sentiment that Griffiths (2007) is trying to convey.

In one sentence, I would say a perfect example of a medical student with exceptional reflective ability whilst demonstrating his genuine concern for his patients by maintaining his focus on the human aspect of the patient role. Griffiths's (2007) reflection has everything that one expects to find in a genuinely caring practitioner. The simple message is that there is no greater care than to demonstrate to patients that we have some understanding of their experience of illness. I used the words *some understanding* instead of *total understanding* as it is doubtful whether this is possible. For example, to say that I fully understand what suffering from schizophrenia is in spite of my clinical and educational experience would be a gross exaggeration. As Walton (1999) states that few illnesses in today's world are as baffling as schizophrenia. The best health care professionals can do is to listen to their patients and involve them in the process of care.

The process of engagement

In order to fully understand the notion of engaging patients in care, it is necessary to highlight some models of care in current use and these include paternalistic, informed, and shared models. The latter seems to embrace the notion of engagement. The paternalistic model promotes the sentiment that health care professionals know best, thus forcing patients towards a passive role. The implication is that health care professionals will make what they consider to be the best treatment decisions for patients without necessarily consulting them. The attitude is one of *I know what is best for you so don't worry you are safe in my hands.* Paternalism, it would seem, is endemic within the British National Health Service (NHS), resulting in an unhealthy dependency, which assumes that health care professionals are the expert treatment decision makers (Coulter, 1999). It is unlikely that paternalistic attitudes in health care provision are confined solely to Britain. However, the implication is that paternalism has no place in the current climate of health care provision regardless of which country one happens to be in. Here, paternalism is portrayed as a negative attribute that one should not even contemplate to embrace in health services. There is no intention here to advocate for paternalism; however, it needs to be pointed out that dismissing it altogether could be seen as *throwing the baby out with the bath water.* Paternalism could be justified in instances where neither patients nor significant others are able to make an autonomous decision. In this instance paternalism could serve to satisfy the needs of patients and those of significant others.

'Patients have grown up-and there's no going back' (Coulter, 1999, p. 719). One can assume from this quote that patients are getting wiser and are no longer perceived as passive recipient of care. In fact, some would argue that they are experts, hence the term 'expert patient'. Conceptualising patients as experts would be seen as a positive move to care. One can't help but to pose the following question, *could expert patient be a mythical concept given the maze of ambiguity in health care settings, roles constraint, and control that result from a perceived or real imbalance of power between professionals and patients?* Moreover, by its very nature, the health care environment can be disempowering to the recipient of care (see Chapter 3). These, one could argue, are further compounded by poor communication among professionals as well as between professionals and patients (see Ley, 1988). Patients can't help but to view health care practitioners, be they doctors, nurses, social workers, occupational therapists, or physiotherapists, as experts. Contemporary philosophies of care seem to suggest that health care professionals should view patients as experts in identifying and expressing their needs. It is debatable whether patients and health care professionals are ready to embrace this new way of thinking. It could be argued that generally, health care professionals, no matter which discipline, are perceived as the experts by themselves and by their patients. The following scenario (based on a personal communication with one of my students) is a case in point to demonstrate one particular patient's perception.

A staff nurse was conducting a drug administration round with a student nurse. Staff nurse was called away during the round; however, prior to leaving, she had asked the student nurse to take some medications to a patient (John). Unfortunately, the student nurse went and gave the medications to a different patient (James). James had no hesitation in taking the medications even though he thought it was strange because the tablets were different to those that he usually takes. Realising the error, the staff nurse then informed James who was not surprised at all. However, when questioned as to why he had taken the medications James said *I was going to ask if my tablets have been changed but then I trusted you to know more than me. I thought the doctor might have changed them without telling me. So I took them.*

It would seem clear that although one may wish to think of patients as experts, it does not necessarily follow that the latter feels and behaves as such. In fact, it could be said that based on the above scenario James was blindly trusting of the student nurse by virtue of her professional role. For James, the student nurse was perceived as more of an expert than him. The student nurse on her part had implicitly assumed that James would query nursing or medical practice. Both parties believe the other to be the expert and the outcome was one extra night in hospital for James, a precautionary measure in response to the wrong medication being administered. The student nurse was left with the guilt of knowing she made a mistake that could have been much more serious than it turned out to be. We can deduce from this that getting to know patients is one of the fundamental principles underpinning health care delivery. The implication is that if health care professionals and patients develop a good relationship with one another then perhaps patients could truly be partners in care. This means going beyond knowing their names and into the realm of understanding who they are, how they feel, and what they think about the changes in their health status.

The British Government does acknowledge paternalism in The NHS as a fact and states that the relationship between service and patients is too hierarchical and paternalistic, thus reflecting the values of 1940s public services (NHS Plan, 2000). Partnership, therefore, is not a characteristic of the paternalistic model. By contrast, the informed model encourages partnership between health care professionals and patients. This, however, is based on what Charles, Whelan, and Gafni (1999) call a division of labour. For example, in relation to information exchange,

> the doctor leads and the communication is one way, from doctor to patient. The doctor communicates to the patient information on all relevant treatment options and their benefits and risks. The amount and type of information communicated includes, at a minimum, sufficient information to enable the patient to make an informed treatment decision.
>
> (Charles, Whelan, & Gafni 1999, p. 781)

The attitude portrayed in this instance is one of *I will provide you with all the information you need but you know what is best for you. Therefore you have to make your own decision.* One of the weaknesses of the informed model is that it can induce a sense of isolation on the part of patients because there is no way of validating their decision except of course after the event.

The shared model, which for the benefit of this discussion is referred to as the engagement model, suggests shared participation in all aspects of care with the principal theme resting on shared or joint decision-making. Charles, Whelan, and Gafni (1999) see decision-making as an iterative process that involves exchange of information, deliberation or discussion of treatment preferences, and deciding on the treatment to implement. Moreover, information exchange can be explored from the following perspectives: flow, direction, type, and amount of information exchanged. Engagement, in its purest form, therefore, involves a two-way process that involves exchange of information between health care practitioner and patient throughout the caring process. The attitude displayed by the professionals is one of *you are not on your own, let's talk and we both can decide what's best for you.*

According to Charles, Gafni, and Whelan (1997)[2] shared decision-making has the following the characteristics.

- At least two participants are involved and these are health care professional and patient. However, it is not unknown to have more than two participants, for example, there may be more than one health care professional in such instances where more than one discipline are involved and these may include doctors, nurses, physiotherapists, occupational therapists, psychologists, and so on. Similarly, patients on their part may wish significant others to be involved. 'The involvement of family members in treatment decision-making may be particularly important with serious illness because of the stress engendered by the diagnosis, the uncertain outcome, and the potentially major impact of the illness trajectory and treatment management on other family members' (Charles, Gafni, & Whelan, 1997, p. 685). Involvement of significant others in the care can add a different dimension to the interaction in that patients may not feel as vulnerable as they would have otherwise felt if they were on their own. Moreover, significant others could take on the role of gathering, recording, and relaying information, or they may prompt the patient to ask relevant questions.

- Both health care professional and patient participate in the process of treatment decision-making. This is not to say that every patient would want to participate in the decision-making process. For example, Degner and Sloan (1992) found that the majority of patients who were newly diagnosed with cancer said they would prefer their physicians to make treatment decisions on their behalf. However, the most popular first choice of patients was that they prefer their doctors to make the final decision about which treatment will be used but that their (patients) opinions should be considered seriously. Interestingly, 51% of the patients in Degner and Sloan's (1992) study wanted their doctor and family to share the responsibility for decision-making if they were too ill to participate. This would appear to reinforce the need to involve significant others in the relationship. Charles, Gafni, and Whelan (1997) raise an important issue in instances where patients may opt for a passive role simply because adopting an active stance may not bode well with health care practitioners. 'No matter how much the patient wants to participate, if the physician is not willing, then shared decision-making will not occur. Similarly, if the physician is willing but the patient is not, then the process will not be shared' (Charles, Gafni, & Whelan, 1997, p. 686).

- Information sharing is a prerequisite to shared decision-making. It would seem obvious that without this *sharing of information* there would be no foundation for the process of engagement to take place. The very essence of shared decision-making is that both health care professional and patient have information to share. However, sometimes neither party knows what information to share and how much information they want from each other. Patients on their part may think health care professionals want information that is only related to their complaint. Health care professionals on their part may feel that patients will only need to know the basics. Both parties therefore must make their individual needs clear to one another and only then shared information will make a difference to decision-making.

A treatment decision is made where both health care professional and patient are in agreement. This would be seen as the best scenario because both parties are in agreement about the treatment option. However, as Charles, Gafni, and Whelan (1997) state, 'this does not mean that both parties are necessarily convinced that this is the best possible treatment for this patient, but rather that both endorse it as the treatment to implement' (p. 688). A health care professional may feel an alternative approach would have been much more appropriate but given that the patient has expressed his or her preference for different treatment leaves the former with little choice but to respect the values of the latter. The crucial issue is that both parties share the responsibility for the outcome of their negotiation.

A model of care and relationship building

Care can be seen as a multifaceted word, for example, it could mean 'serious attention', 'caution', 'protection', or 'look after yourself' as implied in the phrase 'be careful'. From health professionals' perspective care is taken to mean a therapeutic intervention between professionals and those in helping relationships. The term 'intervention' suggests 'an identifiable piece of verbal and/or non-verbal behaviour that is part of the practitioner's service to the client' (Heron, 1990, p. 3). The phrase *therapeutic intervention* represents any activity on the part of health care professionals that enhances a person's growth, development, and personal autonomy. It should be stressed that the emphasis is on *any activity that enhances the health and welfare* of the patients. It would be wrong therefore to assume that any activity on the part of the health care professional[3] is caring. Whatever criteria we choose to imply *care*, one thing is certain and that is *a caring activity* needs to be underpinned by the right attitude in the hands of a knowledgeable and skilled practitioner. Moreover, in order to engage someone effectively in a helping relationship, health care professionals would need to have the interest of that person at heart. This means that as health care professionals, we need to engage with our patients[4] and get to know them in order to help them to be active in their own care.

Figure 9.1 shows a universal model of care integrating the ideas of Peplau (1988) and Rogers (1961) in an attempt to address the needs of individuals, from the point of contact with health care professionals (entry) to leaving health care services (exit). This model serves as a template upon which the ensuing discussion is based.

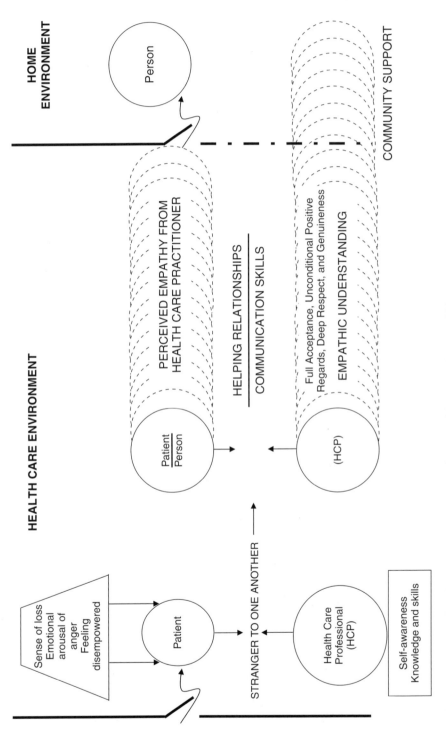

Figure 9.1 A model for care: combining the ideas of Rogers (1961) and Peplau (1988).

Health care professional and patient: Stranger to one another

Peplau (1952) describes the notion of stranger as an encounter between two individuals where neither party is acquainted with one another. Imagine that you are not feeling well (physical or psychological discomfort) and have to be admitted into hospital. When you arrive to your designated ward the first discipline you will most likely encounter is nursing and its practitioners (nurses). It could be said that at this instance the only common knowledge that you share with one another is that you both know that *you* are not well and that something needs to be done to help you recover. The nurses on their part will have the advantage of knowing your name, date of birth, and brief nature of your complaint. You, on the other hand, will know the name of the nurse if and when he or she introduces himself or herself to you (personal experience suggests that nurses don't always introduce themselves to patients although this has not been validated by research). How they introduce themselves to you will most likely lead you to formulate an impression of them. However, your role schema (see Chapter 7) of nurses will dictate your impression of the particular nurse you have encountered. Peplau (1952) advises that it is worthwhile bearing in mind that patients' role schema of nurses is culturally defined and as such will most likely influence their perception. For example, whilst in hospital, one would expect to be in the company of people who have one's interest at heart. This implies that practitioners' verbal, non-verbal, and paralanguages need to be congruent with one another. As health care professionals, therefore, we would need to think carefully what we want to say and how we will need to say it. As Peplau (1952) notes that sometimes health care professionals can feel harassed by their situation to such an extent that it leads to a most inappropriate remark that may be detrimental to the practitioner–patient relationship. Moreover, conveying the impression that suggests *we were not expecting you* can have similar detrimental effect to the relationship. Patients' first impression of the health care practitioner is extremely important because it can lead to primacy effect, as a process whereby the impression people have in the first instance causes them to interpret subsequent behaviour in a manner consistent with how they saw it in the first place. First impression is not always accurate and as Aronson, Wilson, and Akert (1997) state, it is not particularly groundbreaking news to conclude that the longer people get to know one another, the better they get to know each other. However, it could be argued that in health care settings, time is not a luxury afforded to the practitioner to try and change a patient's first impression if this happens to be negative at the first point of contact. Therefore, it is important to convey a positive impression in the first instance. Exercise 3 is an attempt at translating self-knowledge to clinical practice.

EXERCISE 3

Given that you are in the patient role, make a list of how you would like the nurse to behave towards you during this first encounter with him or her.

Reference is made to nurses purely for convenience but issues arising from first impression can be translated to almost any discipline, for example doctors, audiologist, psychologist, and so on. It could be said that often health care professionals dot not see themselves as strangers to patients by virtue of their own comfort based on the familiarity with their environment and its rules and regulations. However, the fact remains that at an interpersonal level they are still strangers to patients. Exercise 4 encourages reflection of self.

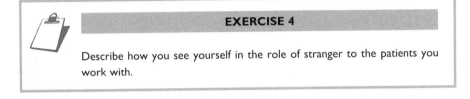

EXERCISE 4

Describe how you see yourself in the role of stranger to the patients you work with.

Partners in care and the helping relationship

According to Peplau (1952), regardless of whom the players are, there is a guiding set of principles that underpins the behaviour of health care practitioners and that is 'respect and positive interest accorded a stranger is at first nonpersonal and includes the same ordinary courtesies that are accorded to a new guest who has been brought into any situation' (p. 44). The implication for practitioners is to accept patients as they are and treat them as people regardless of their role. This means that the barriers that the stranger role poses need to be eliminated to enable the helping relationship to develop. Exercise 5 encourages the use of theoretical knowledge to guide clinical practice.

EXERCISE 5

You might want to explore ways whereby barriers created by the stranger role can be eliminated.

According to Rogers (1967), a helping relationship is 'a relationship in which at least one of the parties has the intent of promoting the growth, development, maturity, improved functioning, improved coping with life of the other' (p. 40). One could safely assume that the party with the intent of promoting growth in the other is the helper. Henceforth, the helper will be referred to as the practitioner or health care professional and the one being helped is the patient. It could be argued that communication skills are important to this helping relationship. However, it would seem that nothing could be more important than the practitioner's attitude in that helping relationship. Having reviewed the works of Heine (1950), Quinn (1950), and Dittes (1957), Rogers (1967) concludes that it is the attitudes and feelings of the therapists rather than their theoretical orientation that is important. This sentiment could be generalised to any health care practitioner. Moreover, it is the way practitioners and their procedures are perceived that makes a difference to patients. For example, only when patients perceive a positive attitude on the part of practitioners that the former will feel the therapeutic effect of the relationship. Rogers (1992) believes that certain core conditions are crucial for change to take place in patients. For the benefit of this discussion, change is taken to mean the process of recovery. Some of these conditions include **F**ull **A**cceptance, **U**nconditional **P**ositive **R**egard, **D**eep **R**espect, **G**enuineness, and **E**mpathy on the part of practitioners. From what Rogers (1992) wrote, it would seem that practitioners would need to go beyond experiencing these conditions and into communicating these feelings and attitudes to their patients. Practitioners would need to be transparent to a point where full acceptance and empathy are reflected in their behaviour, hence the notion of perceived empathy from health care professionals (see Figure 9.1). The ensuing discussion will focus on each of the above mentioned conditions. However, it needs to be pointed out that there are some overlapping sentiments in all these conditions.

Full acceptance

Full acceptance could be seen as the very essence of the caring process and implies a willingness to see the world as perceived by the patient. Davis and Fallowfield (1991) believe acceptance to be a fundamental attitude of assuming the importance of the patient's view and recognising it as such, if only temporarily, the intrinsic truth regardless of the reality. Accepting patients for who they are, implicitly carries the sentiment that this relationship is not between a healthy person and a sick person but instead 'between someone who has delved into his or her own psyche and has come out of this experience not only unscathed but enhanced, and as a result has established an ongoing dialogue with his or her unconscious, and someone who has not undergone this voyage' (Kaufmann, 1989, p. 139). One can deduce from the notion of acceptance that practitioners should not consider themselves superior to patients. Rogers (1967) describes the experience of acceptance as highly rewarding. However, he does recognise the complexity of this task and whether or not one can fully accept another depends on the extent to which one is prepared to confront oneself as exemplified by Rogers (1967, pp. 20–21) in the following questions.

> Can I really permit another person to feel hostile toward me? Can I accept his anger as a real and legitimate part of himself? Can I accept him when he views life and its problems in a way quite different from mine? Can I accept him when he feels very positively toward me, admiring me and wanting to model himself after me?

Interestingly, Rogers believes that people have a tendency to think that every other person must feel and think the same as they do. The implication therefore is that we generally don't believe difference and diversity exist because of our expectation that everyone is similar. This belief could not be further from the truth; and difference and diversity are the very essence of what it takes to be human and only when these are recognised and acknowledged as being real can full acceptance hope to play its part in any relationship. The notion of relationship building and acceptance are aptly captured in the following quote.

> Each person is an island unto himself, in a very real sense; and he can only build bridges to other islands if he is first of all willing to be himself and permitted to be himself. So I find that when I can accept another person, which means specifically accepting the feelings and attitudes and beliefs that he has a real and vital part of him, then I am assisting him to become a person.
>
> (Rogers, 1967, p. 21)

The discussion thus far has focused on what could be described as *acceptance of others*. A further dimension of full acceptance is the *acceptance of self*, which can be as complex as acceptance of others. The idea of *can I accept myself for who I am* is significant in relationship building because it is a prerequisite to accepting others. For example, *how is it possible to accept others for who they are when I can't accept myself for who I am?* Moreover, building a relationship with another person has as its starting point building relationship with self. Rogers (1967) states, 'if I can form a helping relationship to myself – if I can be sensitively aware of and acceptant toward my own feelings – then the likelihood is great that I can form a helping relationship toward another' (p. 51). Interestingly, Kelly (1969) notes that most of us have about as much trouble living with ourselves as we have living with other people. This sentiment is validated by Rogers (1967), who recognises the difficult nature of acceptance of self and admits to have never fully achieved. However, he adds that realising this to be his task

> has been most rewarding because it has helped me to find what has gone wrong with interpersonal relationships which have become snarled and to put them on a constructive track again. It has meant that if I am to facilitate the personal growth of others in relation to me, then I must grow, and while this is often painful it is also enriching.
>
> (Rogers, 1967, p. 51)

Ellis (1977) makes self-acceptance appear so simple by stating that we should fully and unconditionally accept ourselves whether or not we behave intelligently, correctly, or competently and whether or not other people approve or love us. It could be argued that reality may portray a totally different picture in that self-acceptance does not come naturally to everyone.

It is not difficult to imagine why the concept of acceptance can be so complex when we consider the contradictory messages that we have to grapple with in every day life. It may well be that we are responsible for 'creating one kind of society and then lay down rules designed for another' (Kelly, 1969, p. 211).[5] For example, industrialisation and progress made in science especially in the field of transport has meant that people are able to jet from one country to another with reasonable ease. As long as such facilities exist it's reasonable to expect people to make use of them and at that in growing numbers.

However, the tide is beginning to turn and because of fears surrounding global warming there is an attempt to discourage people to use theses facilities. It would not be surprising to see, in future, air travellers stigmatised as outcasts as is the case with smokers. The tobacco industry (indirectly encouraged by the government through taxation to boost the economy) used glowing advertisements to entice the public into a false sense of esteem. Contemporary attitude seems to have taken a U-turn when it is no longer fashionable or 'cool' to engage in these habits. It would seem that smokers are being isolated from the rest of the community because of the numerous venues that prohibit smoking. Moreover, tobacco advertising is now banned from the media. It is not intended here to advocate for smoking, however, this type of 'imposed' isolation stands to make self-acceptance much more difficult for those who engage in the habit.

Unconditional positive regard

Unconditional positive regard is closely related to acceptance of others and suggests 'a warm, positive and acceptant attitude toward what is the client' (Rogers, 1967, p. 62). Moreover, it involves health care professionals' genuine willingness to accept patients regardless of their feelings, experiences, and behaviour. According to Raskin and Rogers (1989), the nature of being human suggests that we freely rely on the evidence of our own senses for making value judgement as opposed to what others feel we ought or should do. Rogers (1951) used the term 'organismic valuing process' to imply that infants evaluate each experience in terms of how it makes them feel and whether or not this experience enhances their sense of self. If our organismic experience is congruent with that of our self-experience, psychological adjustment is believed to take place. Moreover, psychological adjustment is contingent on unconditional positive regard. Psychological maladjustment is said to result from incongruence between organismic experience and self-experience. For example, ignoring or denying one's own feeling to conform with what one *ought* or *should* do leads to what Rogers (1951) termed introjected values that are laden with conditions of worth. To live life burdened by introjected values means that one is merely acting out a script written by others thus real self is not able to take its place in one's life. Take a look at Table 9.1, no doubt you could add to this list.

There is no doubt that condition of worth serves to deny people of their true existence. Rogers (1959) sees unconditional positive regard as one of the necessary conditions for change to occur. However, two questions spring to mind in relation to the practical application of unconditional positive regard.

1. *How realistic is it to expect unconditional positive regard from health care professionals?*

2. *Are we asking for something that contradicts one's feeling in the face of adversity?*

Let's try and explore both these questions in the context of Exercise 6.

Table 9.1 The source of introjected values

No.	Introjected values	Source
1.	I should always be strong and not show my feelings	Because my parents believe that showing one's feeling is a sign of weakness
2.	I should always be successful in my exams	Because my parents have no respect for losers
3.	I should always marry into my own kind	Because of my parents' beliefs
4.	I should always comply with other people's wishes	Because my teacher says it isn't polite to refuse
5.	I should never be serious in a relationship	Because my friends think it isn't 'cool'

Based on Rogers, C. R. (1951). *Client-Centred Therapy: Its Current Practice, Implications, and Theory.* Boston: Houghton Mifflin Company.

EXERCISE 6

A 54-year-old man is admitted to your unit following an unsuccessful suicidal attempt. His medical diagnosis is that of depression. He appears to be pleasant and co-operative on admission but insists that 'you should not waste your time on me as I deserve to die because I have been a bad person'. Describe your feeling and thinking in relation to your ability to offer 'unconditional positive regard'?

It is most likely that 'you should not waste your time on me, as I deserve to die because I have been a bad person' will be treated as a delusional thought. Therefore, one may feel that 'here is a man who is in great need of help' and will most likely offer it contrary to his own self-worth. Your warm, positive and acceptant attitude towards this man is deemed to be justified. However, let's add a twist to this particular scenario (see Exercise 7).

EXERCISE 7

New information has come to light in the form of a court report that gives explicit detail about how this same man has been systematically abusing his two children, a girl of 10 and a boy of 8.

What is your position on this notion of 'unconditional positive regard' now?

This is a very difficult situation to have to face; however, it does put to the test one's ability to adopt an attitude of unconditional positive regard that would have been much easier to adopt if only this man was truly delusional. Could it be that by the very definition of organismic valuing experience and as health care professionals, we are being asked to introject Rogers' philosophies into our systems despite the fact that these may not lead to growth in self? For Rogers (1967), unconditional positive regard is one of the essential conditions for a therapeutic relationship. So what then if one is unable to offer this characteristic in a relationship? Interestingly, Mearns and Thorne (1999) state that whenever practitioners sense an inability to hold an attitude of unconditional positive regard towards their clients they should pay much more attention to empath-ising with them. Empathy would seem to be another problem in the context of our given scenario and this begs the question, *how does one empathise with a parent who has abused his own children given that by nature of role the former is meant to protect the latter?* No attempt will be made here to answer this question except to point out that according to Ellis (1959), neither unconditional positive regard nor empathy is seen as prerequisite for promoting growth in another individual. However, staying with the concept of unconditional positive regard, it is interesting to note the significance of the introduction of new information to whether or not practitioners hold an attitude of unconditional positive regard towards their client. The answer would clearly rest with being human and prac-titioners are just as human as patients. For some of us, therefore, it may be much more difficult to show congruence in a relationship.

The notion of congruence suggests an element of being true to oneself. According to Rogers (1967), the practitioner is in a state of congruence with self when he 'is what he is, when in the relationship with his client he is genuine and without "front" or façade, openly being the feelings and attitudes which at that moment are flowing in him' (p. 61). Unconditional positive regard and congruence are related to one another in that the existence of one facilitates the development of the other (Mearns & Thorne, 1999). Moreover, Mearns and Thorne (1999) see the lack of congruence to be a symptom of difficulties in accepting and trusting the client. Reflecting on the scenario in Exercise 6, it could be argued that there is a clear case for non-acceptance and non-trusting of this particular patient. However, there is something to be said about the role that we have chosen to undertake as health care professionals and this means delivering a non-prejudice and non-discriminatory service. Moreover, Barret-Lennard (1998) states that to be unconditionally responsive to the experiencing person does not mean accepting all their behaviour and certainly does not implying condoning everything they do. One can deduce from this an element of being accepting of the person and not necessarily his or her behaviour. This leads to another question that you may wish to consider, *is it possible for you to accept a person and not his or her behaviour given that as a general rule person and behaviour come as a complete package?*

Deep respect

Deep respect overlaps with acceptance and unconditional positive regard. In fact, Patterson (1985) uses unconditional positive regard and respect as one and the same thing. In being fully accepting of someone and without any precondition one is conveying, implicitly, an attitude of respect. According to Rogers,

> if the therapist holds within himself attitudes of deep respect and full acceptance for this client as he is, and similar attitudes toward the client's potentialities for dealing with himself and his situations; if these attitudes are suffused with a sufficient warmth, which transforms them into the most profound type of liking or affection for the core of the person; and if a level of communication is reached so that the client can begin to perceive that the therapist understands the feelings he is experiencing and accepts him at the full depth of that understanding, then we may be sure that the process is already initiated.
>
> (Rogers, 1967, p. 75)

Before exploring the concept of respect further Exercise 8 may be useful.

EXERCISE 8

Complete the following sentence:
For me respect is . . .

For some, respect is earned and for others respect is something that one is duty bound to afford onto others by virtue of being human. Respecting someone because he or she happens to be human would not sit well with most people because this would imply respecting, for example, someone who abuses children. Moreover, the word respect itself would be so thinly diluted that it could be worthless (Middleton, 2006). The implication is that respect needs to be taken in the context of location instead of personification. That means people should engage in a mutual exchange of respect. However, from a health care perspective, each professional discipline is guided by its own code of ethics where respect for patients is deemed to be of extreme significance. The principal sentiment underpinning most of these statements of intent is that health care professionals are required to recognise and acknowledge the needs and interests of their patients before any therapeutic intervention. This therefore will serve to situate our discussion on respect.

Reflecting on Exercise 8, some of your answers may range from *respect is to feel that I am being listened to without being interrupted* to *being allowed to make a choice without feeling pressured*. Wright, Holcombe, and Salmon (2004) found that doctors communicated respect in two principal ways. These are addressing the patient on the same level and giving the patient the option. At these two levels, therefore, denial of respect could be seen as non-therapeutic because it could serve to hinder growth, development, and personal autonomy. Treating patients with dignity is usually a sign that they are being afforded respect. However, the 'vision of an elderly man in ill-fitting, ill-matching hospital pyjamas being addressed as "love", "pet" or "sweetheart" and under public interrogation as to whether or not his bowels have been opened' (Tadd, Bayer, & Dieppe, 2002, p. 2) is unlikely to demonstrate respect for that particular individual. Exercise 9 attempts to situate the notion of respect to clinical practice.

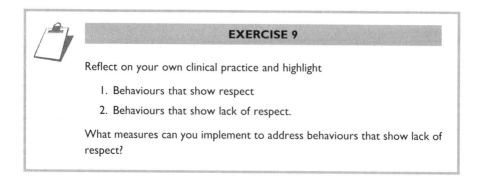

EXERCISE 9

Reflect on your own clinical practice and highlight

1. Behaviours that show respect
2. Behaviours that show lack of respect.

What measures can you implement to address behaviours that show lack of respect?

According to Patterson (1985), the behavioural display of respect can be observed in practitioners' listening skills, in their effort to try and understand their patients, as well as communicating this understanding to the latter. For Rogers (1957), respect for the client is one theme amongst a cluster of conditions that lead to therapeutic growth on the part of the latter. Other conditions include genuineness and empathy.

Genuineness

Genuineness implies being truthful to oneself in a relationship where the practitioner would need to be 'freely and deeply himself, with his actual experience accurately represented by his awareness of himself' (Rogers, 1957, p. 97). Moreover, Rogers argues that practitioners do not necessarily have to exhibit this behaviour in every aspect of their lives, as this may not be possible anyway. This would seem to contrast with Mearns and Thorne (1999) who state that practitioners' ability to be genuine in their therapeutic encounters is related to how genuinely they conduct themselves in social relationships. 'There is something not a little spine-chilling about the counsellor who has the apparent capacity to "turn on" her genuineness at the moment when the therapeutic hour begins, as if congruence were some kind of behavioural technique which can be applied when required' (Mearns & Thorne, 1999, p. 29). This sentiment is validated by Egan (2002) who identified *overemphasising the helping role* as a sign of lack of genuineness. 'Genuine helpers do not take refuge in the role of counsellor. Ideally, relating at deeper levels to others and helping are part of their lifestyles, not roles they put on or take off at will' (Egan, 2002, p. 53). Genuineness with self also applies to behaviour that may not be conducive with the notion of caring. For example, Patterson (1985) posits that genuineness is not always therapeutic in that it is unlikely that those who are highly authoritative and dogmatic will facilitate changes in their patients. This implies that genuineness may not be a necessary condition for therapeutic change to take place. Moreover, Carkhuff and Berenson (1967) conclude that 'while it appears of critical importance to avoid the conscious or unconscious façade of "playing the therapeutic role", the necessity for the therapist's expressing himself fully at all times is not supported' (p. 29). Genuineness it would seem does not necessitate that practitioners always express all of their feelings. As Patterson (1985) states, it only requires that whatever they do express is real and not incongruent with how they are feeling. Moreover, at a minimal level genuineness should not be perceived as being insincere or dishonest. Spontaneity in behaviour is one of the characteristics of genuineness. For example, Egan (2002) states that effective practitioners do not constantly weigh what they say to the patients. Neither do they 'put a number of filters between their inner lives and what they express to others' (Egan, 2002, p. 54). Being genuine does not necessarily mean saying everything that comes to mind. In fact Carkhuff and Berenson (1967) warn that genuineness must not be confused with free license for practitioners to do whatever they choose to do especially if this means freely expressing hostility. The whole emphasis seems to be focused on the idea of not ignoring how one feels during this relationship but to accept that these feelings are real. For example, it would be *true genuineness* on the part of practitioners to be aware that they may not be in the right frame of mind to listen attentively to their patients. For Rogers (1957), when the practitioner 'is not denying these feelings to awareness, but is able freely to be them (as well as being his other feelings), then the condition we have stated is met' (p. 97).

Empathy

Empathy and empathic understanding are discussed in Chapter 1, and in this section the focus is more on conveying empathic understanding to the patient. Empathic understanding, as was presented in Chapter 1, is said to be evident when the practitioner is able to capture the patient's feelings, emotions, and thoughts through his or her words and actions as well as relaying this information to the patient, hence the notion of perceived empathic understanding on the part of the patient (see Figure 9.1). Perceived empathic understanding is also known as interactive empathy in that practitioners are able to sense the emotions of another person and communicate this understanding to them (Natale, 1972). The starting point of interactive empathy is the practitioners' ability to abandon themselves and relive in themselves the emotions and responses of patients. However, according to Katz (1963), it is a matter of common experience that people in general find it more difficult to establish empathy with those who are different and diverse from themselves. The implication is that it may not always be possible to empathise with the other person especially if one has little understanding of how the other person functions. This is particularly relevant where culturally patients are different from practitioners. Cultural empathy will be discussed later in this chapter. According to Katz (1963), 'it is almost impossible for us, if we are men, to empathize with such exclusively feminine experiences as menstruating or giving birth' (pp. 6–7). It is worthwhile reiterating that generally there is a tendency to empathise with those who are familiar to us or whose life situation is most similar to our own (Katz, 1963).

According to Horton (2000), there are four levels of empathy and these are as follows.

1. Perception level relates to what practitioners see or hear from the patient.
2. Affect level emphasises what practitioners feel when they are attentively listening to the patient.
3. Cognition level focuses on what practitioners understand and imagine about the patient's experience.
4. Communication level conveys practitioners' empathic understanding to the patient through verbal behaviour, non-verbal behaviour, and paralanguages. The content of this communication could include practitioners' perception, affect, and cognition. In fact these would form the essence of perceived empathic understanding.

These levels of empathy suggest the depth of understanding achieved by practitioners as well as how these are communicated to the patient. According to Egan (2002, p. 97), the assumption is that practitioners need not only be accurate perceivers but that they should also have the ability to 'weave their perceptions into their dialogues' with their patients. This can be achieved by 'sharing empathic highlights with their clients' (Egan, 2002, p. 97). The term 'highlights' suggests that practitioners' focus is on the principal issues that emerge during the interaction. Egan (2002), like Raskin and Rogers (1989), feels that the response that practitioners offer to patient needs to be much more than paraphrasing or restating. 'If you are truly empathic, if you listen actively, and if you thoughtfully process what you hear, putting what the client says in its proper context, then you do more than paraphrase or restate. There is something of you in your response' (Egan, 2002, p. 97). The implication for health care students therefore is that it is not sufficient to say that *I showed empathy with my patients* instead you will have to let the evidence speak for itself. For example, one should be able to establish your ability to empathise with your patients by the response that you offer them (see Table 9.2 for tendency towards empathic understanding). Obviously, those who have a tendency towards egocentrism will find it much more difficult to empathise with others. Empathy, like these other therapeutic conditions, cannot be switched on and off and depends very much on practitioners' ability to put themselves in the place of their patients as in stepping into their shoes, thus obtaining an inside knowledge that is described as almost first hand (Fliess, 1942).

Egan (2002) offers a simple formula for basic empathic understanding and this consists of practitioners being able to (a) name the correct emotion expressed by the patient (as in recognising the feeling and mood of the patient) and (b) indicate the correct experiences and behaviours that give rise to the feelings (for example, what cues have led to this conclusion). For example:

Patient: *Everything is getting on top of me and no matter how hard I try I feel as if I am getting nowhere.*

Practitioner (naming the correct emotion): *You feel snowed under and helpless.*

Practitioner (indicating the correct experience and behaviour that give rise to the feelings): *And all your efforts seem to be fruitless and you are not seeing the benefit.*

Table 9.2 Some examples of 'tendency towards empathy' and 'tendency towards egocentric thinking'

	Tendency towards empathy	Tendency towards egocentric thinking
1	I feel sad when I see someone in pain	People should learn to cope with their pain and not complain all the time
2	I tend to get emotionally involved with a friend's problem	I find it difficult to understand how my friends could get upset about trivial things
3	I cry sometimes when I watch a sad film	I can't understand why people get so emotionally involved in films
4	Shivers go through my spine when I hear someone receiving bad news	Life has its ups and downs, one needs to accept this as fact

Adapted from Mehrabein, A. and Epstein, N. (1972). A measure of emotional empathy. *Journal of Personality*, 40, 525–543.

Cultural empathy

According to Patterson and Watkins (1996), for empathic understanding to be effective knowledge of the patient group alone is not sufficient. Practitioners will have to be able to apply this knowledge during their interactions with their patients. The implication is that awareness of cultural uniqueness and its significance in the patient's life needs to be recognised and practitioners' subsequent behaviour should be guided by these variables. A view echoed by Ibrahim (1991) who states that 'the ability to convey empathy in a culturally consistent and meaningful manner may be the crucial variable to engage the client. Understanding of client worldviews and cultural identification and having a clearer comprehension of client concerns can greatly facilitate empathic understanding and responding' (p. 18). The problem, however, clearly rests on which paradigm the concept of illness is based upon. For example, if the concept of illness is based on western culture then it follows that the delivery of care will be defined by that particular culture. Empathic understanding becomes problematic because practitioners will be hindered by their own ethnocentrism.[6] According to Sue and Sue (1990), culturally skilled practitioners attempt to be active in the process of understanding the worldview of culturally different patients. Rogers' (1951) position on practitioners' cultural awareness of their clients is reflected in the following quote. 'We fail to see that we are evaluating the person from our own, or from some fairly general, frame of reference, but that the only way to understand his behaviour meaningfully is to understand it as he perceives it himself, just as the only way to understand another culture is to assume the frame of reference of that culture' (Rogers, 1951, p. 494). However, it could be argued that cultural empathy may not always be a necessary condition for therapeutic change to take place. Some would argue that it might in fact hinder the relationship. For example, Usher (1989) posits that empathic understanding may be perceived as offensive in cultures where reservation and inhibition are valued in relationship especially with strangers. Moreover, Patterson and Watkins (1996) state that clinicians can assess cultural-experiential determinants by inquiring along appropriate lines. One prerequisite would, in this instance, be that patients must be prepared to self-disclose to their practitioners. Given that self-disclosure is culturally defined, cultural empathy may not be attainable in some situation.

Cultural empathy leads to what can be described as cultural competence, which requires that practitioners become expert in cultural differences and diversity of patients. A culturally competent health care system is seen as one that acknowledges and incorporates at all levels the importance of culture, assessment of cross-cultural relations, vigilance towards the dynamics that result from cultural differences, expansion of cultural knowledge, and adaptation of services to meet culturally unique needs (Betancourt et al., 2003). This may be a tall order for health care professionals because as Dyche and Zayas (1995) state, it is practically impossible for practitioners to learn the background of every culturally diverse patient. According to Dyche and Zayas (2001), understanding cultural empathy requires clarity about the concept of empathy as it occurs in life and in clinical practice. Subsidiary to cultural empathy is the notion of cross-cultural receptivity. 'Receptive listeners prefer to experience and describe another's world rather than to define or assess it' (Dyche & Zayas, 2001, p. 249). It could be argued therefore that effective cultural empathy could be developed through the skills of listening (see Chapter 8).

Summary

The basic understanding portrayed here is that patients should be recognised and acknowledged first and foremost for being individuals in their own rights. This would then serve as a foundation for the process of engagement where a real partnership with health care professionals develops. This process would initially start with both professionals and patients being strangers to one another. However, relationship building on the part of practitioners is believed to contribute to patients feeling valued during the transition from patienthood to personhood. Practitioners on their part should communicate empathic understanding, thus portraying a real attempt at therapeutic intervention. An intervention can only be considered therapeutic when it is suffused with full acceptance, unconditional positive regard, deep respect, and genuineness in helping to promote growth, development, and independence on the part of the patient. Two principal barriers pose a threat to the notion of engaging patients in their own care and these are professionals who may choose not to involve patients in the decision-making process and patients themselves who for their own reasons may not wish to be involved. This to some extent makes the whole concept of engagement complex. The proposed model, underpinned by practitioners' skills, knowledge, and attitude that is conducive to the notion of care, attempts to humanise the helping process.

References

Aronson, E., Wilson, T. D., and Akert, R. M. (1997). *Social Psychology*. New York: Longman.

Barret-Lennard, G. T. (1998). *Carl Rogers' Helping System: Journey and Substance*. London: Sage.

Betancourt, J., Green, A. R., Carrillo, J. E., and Ananeh-Firempong II, O. (2003). Defining cultural competence: a practical framework for addressing racial/ethnic disparities in health and health care. *Public Health Reports*, 118, 293–302.

Carkhuff, R. R. and Berenson, B. G. (1967). *Beyond Counselling and Therapy*. New York: Holt, Rinehart, and Winston, Inc.

Charles, C., Gafni, A. and Whelan, T. (1997). Shared decision-making in the medical encounter: what does it mean? (Or it takes at least two to tango). *Social Sciences Medicine*, 44(5), 681–692.

Charles, C., Whelan, T., and Gafni, A. (1999). What do we mean by partnership in making decisions about treatment? *British Medical Journal*, 319, 780–782.

Coulter, A. (1999). Paternalism or partnership? *British Medical Journal*, 319, 719–720.

Davis, H. and Fallowfield, L. (1991). Counselling and communication in Health Care. Chichester, New York, and Brisbane: John Wiley and Sons.

Degner, L. F. and Sloan, J. A. (1992). Decision making during serious illness: what role do patients really want to play? *Journal of Clinical Epidemiology*, 9, 941–950.

Dittes, J. (1957). Galvanic skin response as a measure of patients' reaction to therapist permissiveness. *Journal of Abnormal Psychology*, 18, 191–196.

Dyche, L. and Zayas, L. H. (1995). The value of curiosity and naiveté for the cross-cultural psychotherapist. *Family Process*, 34, 389–399.

Dyche, L. and Zayas, L. H. (2001). Cross-cultural empathy and training the contemporary psycho-therapist. *Clinical Social Work Journal*, 29(3), 245–258, Fall.

Egan, G. (2002). *The Skilled Helper: A Problem-Management and Opportunity-Development Approach to Helping*. Belmont: Brooks/Cole.

Ellis, A. (1959). Requisite conditions for basic personality change. *Journal of Counselling Psychology*, 23, 538–540.

Ellis, A. (1977). The basic clinical theory of rationale-emotive therapy. In A. Ellis and R. Grieger (eds.), *A Handbook of Rationale-Emotive Therapy* (pp. 3–34). New York: Springer.

Fliess, R. (1942). The metapsychology of the analyst. *The Psychoanalytic Quarterly*, 11(2), 211–227.

Griffiths, B. W. (2007). Uncomfortable experience. *SBMJ*, 15, 35.

Hart, N. (1985). *The Sociology of Health and Medicine: Themes and Perspectives in Sociology*. Ormskirk: Causeway Press Limited.

Heine, R. W. (1950). *A Comparison of Patients' Reports on Psychotherapeutics Experience with Psycho-analytic, Nondirective, and Alderrian Therapists*. Unpublished doctoral dissertation. University of Chicago.

Heron, J. (1990). *Helping the Client: A Creative Practical Guide*. London: Sage.

Horton, I. (2000). Therapeutic skills and clinical practice: structuring. In C. Feltham and I. Horton (eds.), *Handbook of Counselling and Psychotherapy* (pp. 111–122). London, Thousand Oaks, and New Delhi: Sage Publications.

Ibrahim, F. A. (1991). Contribution of cultural worldview to generic counselling and development. *Journal of Counselling and Development*, 70, 13–19.

Katz, R. L. (1963). *Empathy: Its Nature and Uses*. London: The Free Press of Glencoe.

Kaufmann, Y. (1989). Analytic psychotherapy. In R. J. Corsini and D. Wedding (eds.), *Current Psychotherapies* (pp. 118–152). Itasca: F. E. Peacock Publishers, Inc.

Kelly, G. (1969). Humanistic methodology in psychological research. In B. Maher (ed.), *Clinical Psychology and Personality: Selected Papers of George Kelly*. London: Wiley.

Ley, P. (1988). *Communicating with Patients: Improving Communication, Satisfaction and Compli-ance*. London: Croom Helm.

McKevitt, C. and Morgan, M. (1997). Anomalous patients: the experiences of doctors with illness. *Sociology of Health and Illness*, 19(5), 644–667.

Mearns, D. and Thorne, B. (1999). *Person-Centred Counselling in Action*. London, Thousand Oaks, and New Delhi: Sage Publications.

Mehrabein, A. and Epstein, N. (1972). A measure of emotional empathy. *Journal of Personality*, 40, 525–543.

Middleton, D. (2006). Introduction. *Research Publication*, 12, 1–7.

Natale, S. (1972). *An Experiment in Empathy*. Slough: National Foundation for Educational Research in England and Wales.

NHS Plan (2000). *A Plan for Investment, a Plan for Reform*. London: HMSO.

Parsons, T. (1951). *The Social System*. Glenco: Free Press.

Patterson, C. H. (1985). Respect (Unconditional Positive Regrad). *The Therapeutic Relationship* (pp. 59–63). Monterey: Brooks/Cole. Available at http://www.sageofasheville.com/pub_ downloads/RESPECT_(UNCONDITIONAL_POSITIVE_REGARD).pdf.

Patterson, C. H. and Watkins, C. E. (1996). *Theories of Psychotherapy* (5th edn.). New York: HarperCollins.

Peplau, H. E. (1952/1988). *Interpersonal Relations in Nursing*. London: Macmillan Education.

Quinn, R. D. (1950). *Psychotherapists' Expressions as an Index to the Quality of Early Therapeutic Relationships*. Unpublished doctoral dissertation. University of Chicago.

Raskin, N. J. and Rogers, C. R. (1989). Person centered therapy. In R. J. Corsini and D. Wedding (eds.), *Current Psychotherapies* (pp. 155–194). Itasca: F. E. Peacock Publishers, Inc.

Rogers, C. R. (1951). *Client-Centred Therapy: Its Current Practice, Implications, and Theory*. Boston: Houghton Mifflin Company.

Rogers, C. R. (1957). The necessary and sufficient conditions of therapeutic personality change. *Journal of Consulting Psychology*, 21, 95–103.

Rogers, C. R. (1959). A theory of therapy, personality and interpersonal relationships, as developed in the client-centered framework. In S. Koch (ed.), *Psychology: A study of Science* (pp. 184–256). New York: McGraw Hill.

Rogers, C. R. (1961). *On Becoming a Person: A Therapist's View of Psychotherapy*. Boston: Houghton Mifflin.

Rogers, C. R. (1967). *On Becoming a Person: A Therapist's View of Psychotherapy*. London: Constable.

Rogers, C. R. (1992). The necessary and sufficient conditions of therapeutic personality change. *Journal of Consulting and Clinical Psychology*, 60(6), 827–832.

Russell, S. (1999). An exploratory study of patients' perceptions, memories and experiences of an intensive care unit. *Journal of Advanced Nursing*, 29(4): 783–791.

Sue, D. W. and Sue, D. (1990). *Counselling the Culturally Different: Theory and Practice* (2nd edn.) New York: John Wiley and Sons.

Tadd, W., Bayer, T., and Dieppe, P. (2002). Dignity in health care: reality or rhetoric. *Reviews in Clinical Gerontology*, 12: 1–4.

Usher, C. H. (1989). Recognizing cultural bias in counselling theory and practice: the case of Rogers. *Journal of Multicultural Counselling and Development*, 17, 62–71.

Walton, J. A. (1999). On living with schizophrenia. In I. Madjar and J. A. Walton (eds.), *Nursing and the Experience of Illness: Phenomenology in Practice* (98–122). London and New York: Routledge.

Wright, E. B., Holcombe, C. and Salmon, P. (2004). Doctor's communication of trust, care, and respect in breast cancer: qualitative study. *British Medical Journal*, 328, 864.

Concluding Remarks

An attempt has been made, through a variety of exercises, to show a link between the notion of care and self-awareness on the part of health care professionals. The implication is that self-knowledge serves as a foundation for understanding those people who need to access health care services. The underpinning sentiment of *Self-Awareness in Health Care* is based on the idea that recognising, acknowledging, and perhaps more importantly, accepting patients' felt experience is the first step in the engagement process. Engagement, in its simplest form, suggests involving patients in their own care by affording them opportunities to have a greater say in what happens to them. Admittedly, some patients would jump at these opportunities, while others may prefer to adopt a passive role. The same could be said of health care professionals in that some are happy to embrace the notion of engagement by involving patients in their own care, while others may show resistance by adopting much more of an authoritative role. The process of engagement therefore means that health care professionals need to adopt a patient-centered approach by allowing patients to identify their needs and goals. This means that wherever appropriate, health care professionals should take on a facilitative role in working with patients' needs. However, this does not imply that if a patient is confused, disorientated, and expresses the need not to eat over a period of time he or she is allowed to starve. In circumstances where practitioners have doubt in their patients' cognitive ability then perhaps it is best to allow oneself to be guided by the Ethics of Reciprocity commonly known as the Golden Rule. This suggests that *we do onto others as we would wish them do onto us.* Moreover, commonsense and duty of care suggest that as health care professionals, we would need to intervene by assuming some responsibility to ensure our patients' nutritional needs (or any other needs) are satisfied.

By recognising the transitional process from person to patient, health care professionals may gain a greater insight into patients' felt experience in that illness may result in stress and anxiety, loss and grief, and anger and aggression. By definition, the patient role may be perceived as disempowering because of the potential loss of independence and freedom afforded to healthy individuals. Moreover, by the very nature of health care institutions patients may feel strangers to their new surrounding and its occupants (health care professionals as well as other patients). The health care professional–patient relationship therefore is crucial to the successful transition from patient to autonomous person. This relationship, however, would need to engender therapeutic growth on the part of the patient. Some of the core conditions that would facilitate this therapeutic growth are empathic understanding, acceptance, and prizing of the patient as in offering unconditional positive regards. Theoretically, these skills are easily understood in terms of what they aim to achieve. Their applications to practice may be challenging for some professionals. However, embracing the skills of emotional and social intelligence may help to reduce self-contradiction on the part of practitioners. It is argued that by using information obtained from self-monitoring of own feelings and emotions to guide thinking and actions, practitioners should be in a better position to understand and manage their relationships with patients. The model of care presented in *Self-Awareness in Health Care* emphasises a practitioner–patient relationship whereby the stranger role is transformed to partners in care, thus giving some responsibilities to the patient who may feel much more in control of the way care is delivered.

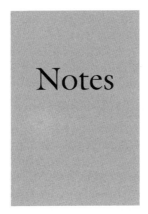

Notes

I Self-awareness

1. Psychological strategies employed by an individual in order to protect him or her from anxiety or internal conflict.

2. They may hold aggressive sexual impulses, but these are deemed to be immoral.

3. This excludes people who due to certain type of mental health problem may not have insight into their health state.

4. See Chapter 4.

2 Stress, vulnerability, and self-awareness

1. See Chapters 6 and 7 for a definition of schema.

2. Identification can be described as the process during which a child takes on the characteristics of a significant other (usually a parent), thus reducing his or her anxieties and internal conflicts.

3 Power, empowerment, and self-awareness in helping relationships

1. Camp Delta in Guantanamo Bay, Cuba: A military-run prison where alleged terrorists are kept.

2. Detail of Milgram's experiment can be found in Milgram (1974).

3. An actor.

4. See http://www.bmj.com/cgi/eletters/323/7310/414.

5. A life-threatening condition of pregnancy that is characterised by high blood pressure and fluid retention.

6. 'Ex parte' a Latin term in a UK legal context meaning 'proceeding brought by one person in the absence of another'.

7. See Chapter 2.

4 Emotion of loss and self-awareness

1. Object can include people, animal, personal possessions, and life styles (careers).

2. See Chapter 1 (Self-Awareness).

3. Disorientation in terms of place, person, and time.

4. Seen as the intensification of grief to the level where the person is overwhelmed, resorts to maladaptive behaviour, or remains interminably in the state of grief without progression of the mourning process towards completion. 'Pathological mourning' involves processes that do not move progressively towards assimilation or accommodation but, instead, lead to stereotyped repetitions or extensive interruptions of healing (Horowitz et al., 1980, p. 1157).

5. Sometimes referred to as inhibited, suppressed, or postponed grief reactions.

6. I highly recommend that you refer to Worden (2003).

7. [of helping] is added in an attempt to link Rogers' sentiment in the context of our discussion.

5 Anger, aggression, and self-awareness

1. It would appear that life preferences are significant to one's level of testosterone. For example, Archer's (2006) conclusion is that high testosterone men devote more time and energy to mating than to parental effort. For a more detail account see Archer (2006).

2. Hoffman (1960, p. 130) offers the following explanation for unqualified power assertion: 'Because of his strong power position, the parent is free to choose influence techniques which, in varying degrees, assert power or attempt to induce the child to change his behaviour voluntarily.... These techniques, exemplified by direct commands, threats, deprivations, and physical force, we refer to as *unqualified power assertion.*'

3. See Baumeister, R. F., Smart, L., and Boden, J. M. (1996). Relation of threatened egotism to violence and aggression: the dark side of high self-esteem. *Psychological Review*, 103, 5–33 and Bushman, B. J. and Baumeister, R. F. (1998). Threatened egotism, narcissism, self-esteem, and direct and displaced aggression: does self-love or self-hate lead to violence? *Journal of Personality and Social Psychology*, 75, 219–229.

4. See Chapter 7 for a detailed discussion of the notion of schema.

5. See Chapter 7 for a detailed discussion on attitude.

6. See 'Frustration–Aggression Hypothesis' as previously discussed in this chapter.

7. Defined as the ability to recall meanings for general and factual information.

6 The use of language and self-awareness

1. PET techniques – does not lose sensitivity and spatial localisation, does not create the din that is a feature of data acquisition in an MR scanner, and can be a less intimidating environment (than going into a MRI magnet).

2. fMRI techniques – combines greater spatial resolution, faster temporal resolution, and no exposure of the patient to radiation.

3. See Chapter 7.

4. See Haffner (1992). We considered this article to be excellent in making clear the importance of 'getting it right' when we are communicating with others.

8 Interpersonal communication and interpersonal skills

1. Survival is taken to mean healthy mental state.

2. There in no intention here to discuss this further; however, you may find wish to refer to Schutz (1966).

3. For a more detailed account of these questions refer to Egan (1977).

9 Engagement and developing relationships

1. Square brackets added to make explicit Griffiths's quote. Moreover, paragraphs have been restructured to fit with the style of this book.

2. In their discussion, Charles, Gafni, and Whelan (1997) refer to physician–patient partnership. I, on the other hand, am generalising this partnership by making reference to any health care professional regardless of discipline.

3. Used interchangeably with practitioner and carer.

4. Used interchangeably with client, service user, one in a helping relationship, and people in need of help.

5. This quote is used in a different context from Kelly's (1969) idea.

6. Ethnocentrism can be defined as the tendency to see the world from the viewpoint of one's own culture.

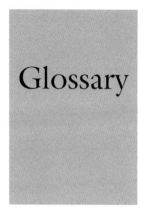

Glossary

Abdicrat	An individual who would prefer to avoid responsibility and power with a tendency to veer towards subordination.
Abnormal grief	A maladaptive response to loss where an individual is not able to move satisfactorily through the grieving stages.
Accommodation	Modification made to the existing schema in order to take on board new information.
Accountability	Having to answer to someone, for example an employer or a professional body.
Acquired vulnerability	This means that people are generally prone to a given illness by virtue of being previously exposed to trauma, disease, family experiences, hostile environment, and so on.
Actor-observer effect	When people make mistakes they are stupid, but when I make a mistake it is because I was distracted.
Aesthetic value	Beauty as something very precious.
Affective aggression	Also known as emotional aggression and seen as violent acts triggered by intense anger.
Affective self	This is the feeling aspect of self and involves emotions.
Aggression	A goal-directed behaviour or response that delivers a negative or aversive stimulus to others with the intent to cause harm.
Alarm stage	The body senses danger.

Alopecia	Loss of hair.
Anger	A natural emotional arousal followed by the thought of attacking.
Angiography	Examination of the blood vessels using x-rays following the injection of a radiopaque substance.
Anhedonia	Inability to experience pleasure from pleasurable events.
Anticipatory grief	Response to the loss object starts before the loss has actually occurred.
Antihypertensive therapy	Treatment to reduce high blood pressure.
Aphasia	Inability to speak.
Aphonia	Loss of voice.
Apnoea	Temporary absence or cessation of breathing.
Assimilate	The taking on of new information.
Assimilation	The act of taking on new information.
Asymmetry	Uneven.
Attachment	A strong emotional bond or tie with an object (thing, people, or animal).
Attitude	A state of readiness organised through experience and influences a person's response to his or her situation.
Attributes	Traits and/or characteristics.
Attribution	The process through which individuals seek to explain why they do what they do.
Authenticity	Genuineness.
Autocrat	An individual who prefers to have control and power in a group.
Autokinetic effect	When a person perceives a fixed point of light shone onto a wall in a darkened room to move.
Autonomy	Self-sufficient or self-dependent and freely choosing.
Aversive stimulus	A negative trigger.
Behavioural script	The way we behave in different context.
Behavioural self	The action that one engages in and this could be verbal and/or non-verbal.
Bereavement	The experience of grieving.
Blame culture	A way of life that favours apportioning blame onto someone else.
Cardiovascular	Relating to the heart and the blood vessels.
Cerebro-vascular disease	This is commonly known as stroke and includes all disorders where an area of the brain is transiently or permanently affected by lack of or reduced blood supply.

Classical conditioning	Two stimuli are repeatedly paired until the presence of one evokes the expectation of the other.
Clostridium difficile	A bacterium of the family Clostridium (the family also includes the bacteria that cause tetanus, botulism, and gas gangrene). It is an anaerobic bacterium (that is, it does not grow in the presence of oxygen) and produces spores that can survive for a long time in the environment.
Cognitive appraisal	This is an evaluative and continuous process that occurs throughout our waking lives where meaning is given to the event its relevance to self is established.
Cognitive dissonance	A condition of conflict or anxiety resulting from inconsistency between beliefs and actions.
Cognitive self	This is also referred to as the mental process of comprehension and includes memory, perception, past experience, expectation, appraisal, attribution, attitude, beliefs, and values. Cognitive self is basically *the thinking aspect of self*.
Cognitive triad	A set of assumptions that suggests a person holding a negative view of self (I am worthless), negative view of the world (this is an awful place to be), and negative view of the future (it can only get worse from here on).
Compliance	Changing our behaviour as a result of a direct request from someone who has no authority over us.
Compulsory detention	Held against one's will.
Confederate	Someone who is in on the plot.
Conformity	Changing one's behaviour in keeping with the behaviour of other group members.
Consciousness	To be aware of the *here and now*.
Conservation	The physical properties of things (amount, size, volume, and weight) remain the same even though their shapes or appearances may change.
Critical period	A stage in development where an organism is at its optimum to learn a new behaviour.
Cultural empathy	Understand people from their own way of life dictated by a set of rules imposed by their societal norm.
Deep respect	Being fully accepting of someone and without any precondition demonstrates an attitude of respect.
Degenerate	Someone who is inefficient due to lack of knowledge.
Delayed grief	The experience of pain usually associated with the loss object at the time of the loss that is not displayed until much later.

Delusion	A false belief strongly held in spite of invalidating evidence.
Democrat	An individual who feels that he or she is a capable, responsible person and therefore does not need to shrink from responsibility or to try constantly to prove how competent he or she really is.
Denial	A way of avoiding or escaping from certain unpleasant realities by behaving as if these have not occurred.
Detachment	Separation as in to be apart.
Diagnosis	Determining the nature and cause of an illness.
Diathesis	A predisposition to a particular illness, which is developed as a consequence of stress.
Disempowerment	A process that encourages social control and dependency on the part of the patient.
Displacement	The shifting of emotion from a situation or object with which it is truly related to another target.
Dispositional attribution	Also known as internal attribution where behaviour is linked directly to the person. For example, I pass my exam because I am clever.
Dizygotic twins	Twins derived from two eggs.
Dyspepsia	Indigestion.
Dysphagia	Difficulty in swallowing.
Economic values	Material gain is important.
Economy or knowledge	Serves to inform.
Egocentric assumptions	The tendency to make attribution based on personal needs or wishes when faced with insufficient information.
Egocentric language	Talking for self or for the pleasure of associating anyone who happens to be present.
Egocentric thinking	An individual can only see it from his or her own perspective.
Ego-defensive	Self-deception.
Electra complex	This is similar phenomenon to Oedipus complex that happens during child development where little girls develop a special kind of affection for their fathers.
Embeddedness	The integration of a stimulus into its environment.
Emotional intelligence	The ability to monitor one's own feeling and emotions to discriminate among them and to use this information to guide one's thinking and actions.
Emotion-focused coping	Energy is spent on regulating the distressing emotions associated with problems.

Empathic listening	Listening in order to understand the other person's point of view.
Empathic understanding	The emotional knowing of another person's feeling.
Engagement	Encourage patients to take an active part in what happens to them when they become ill, to collaborate in their care, and to work in partnership with health care professionals (or) A two-way process that involves exchange of information between health care practitioner and patient throughout the caring process.
Eros	Freudian concept for the instinct of life.
Errors and biases	Misinterpretation of events because these are usually perceived outside the context that which they appear.
Event schemas	Also known as scripts relate to the knowledge about the procedures associated with familiar social situations. For example, we all know what happens at a wedding.
Examplification	Going to great length to show one's dedication to one's job such as working outside the calls of duty.
Exhaustion stage	This is the result of depletion of adaptive energy and could lead to death.
Expressive aphasia	Also known as Broca's aphasia is the inability to speak.
External locus of control	The belief that what happens to individuals is outside of their control as in luck or fate. For example, my destiny is in your hand.
Fistula	An abnormal passage resulting from injury.
Foot-in-the-door technique	Compliance for a larger request is easily achieved when this is preceded by a small request.
Full acceptance	A willingness to recognise and acknowledge patients for whom they are.
Genuineness	Being truthful to oneself in a relationship where individuals would need to be freely and deeply themselves, with their actual experiences accurately represented by their awareness of themselves.
Geographical cure	Moving to a different location in the hope that this will solve the problem
Gesture	Body language that reveals information within the context of a given situation and involves part or parts of the body.
Goal competence	The ability to set goals and anticipate its possible outcome as well as choosing an effective course of action.
Grief	A natural response to the loss object and is displayed emotionally, physically, and socially.

Hallucination	Perception of visual, auditory, tactile, olfactory, or gustatory experiences without any external stimuli but with a compelling sense of their reality.
Hate	An intense negative and undesirable emotion with intent of destructive aggression.
Heart murmur	An abnormal heart condition evidenced by extra sound during the heartbeat cycle when blood goes through the heart and its valves.
Hemiplegia	Paralysis affecting one side of the body.
Hominoids	Belonging to the superfamily Hominoidea that includes apes and humans.
Hostility	A negative attitude towards someone that is reflected in a decidedly unfavourable judgement with a desire for that person to suffer.
Hypertensive	High blood pressure.
Ideas of reference	A delusional belief where individuals feel that others are talking about them.
Imagined loss	Misinterpretation or false perception of being separated from one's object of attachment.
Impersonal communication	The individuality and uniqueness of individuals are not recognised and are treated as objects or labels.
Inborn vulnerability	This means that people are generally predisposed to a given illness by virtue of their heredity (nature).
Inclusion	The need to be with people and to be alone, to have enough contact to avoid loneliness, and enough aloneness to avoid enmeshment and enjoy solitude.
Incubation period	The period of time required for the development of symptoms of a disease after infection.
Ingratiation	Trying to get in other people's good books.
Instinct	Unlearned pattern of behaviour.
Instrumental aggression	Aggressive acts with the intent to cause harm but with no malice intended (as in using aggressive behaviour for self-defence).
Internal locus of control	The belief that individuals are personally responsible for what happens to them, for example, my destiny is in my own hands.
Interpersonal communication	Interpersonal communication is said to take place when people treat one another as unique individuals, regardless of the context in which the interaction occurs or the number of people involved.

Interpersonal skill	The ability to comprehend the nature of social interactions, to be able to make an accurate judgement of the behaviour of others, as well as being able to act in a way that enhances relationships.
Interpersonal styles	The general ways of behaving in company of others.
Interpretive competence	The ability to make an accurate judgement of what is going on with another person as well as what is going on within oneself.
Intimidation	Use of threat to show who is in charge.
Intrapersonal communication	The exchange of information within oneself. This involves cognitive and emotive selves.
Introjection	A process whereby an individual takes on the values or personal attributes of a significant other and behaves as though these are really his or her own.
I-self	Also referred to as the knower is the observation and self-recording processes that generate the knowledge about self.
Language acquisition device	A device in the brain that converts body of utterances into grammatical competence.
Law of effect	If a particular behaviour is rewarded it will most likely be repeated whereas a behaviour that is followed by discomfort will not.
Learned helplessness	This is a psychological state that frequently results when events are perceived as uncontrollable, the resulting belief is that action on the individual's part is futile.
Loss	An emotion that is aroused as a result of separation from an object of attachment.
Lumbar puncture	The insertion of a needle in the lumbar region of the back to withdraw spinal fluid.
Magnitude	Extent or length one is prepared to go to.
Maladaptive behaviour	Undesirable and socially unacceptable behaviour that interferes with the acquisition of desired skills or knowledge.
Mental defence mechanisms	Psychological strategies employed by people in order to protect themselves from anxiety or internal conflict.
Me-self	The knowledge that we have about ourselves such as the sum of all that we call ours.
Message competence	The ability to speak a language that other people can understand and respond to.

Methicillin-resistant *Staphylococcus Aureus*	This is also known as the 'superbug'. It belongs to the *Staphylococcus aureus* family of germs. *Staphylococcus aureus* is a very common cause of bacterial infections, such as boils, carbuncles, infected wounds, deep abscesses, and bloodstream infection.
Monotropy	The principal attachment figure that is perceived to provide the most comfort and security.
Monozygotic twins	Twins that develop from a single fertilised ovum.
Morpheme	Smallest unit of meaningful sound.
Mourning	The period during which grief response is displayed.
Myopia	Short-sightedness.
Necrotic tissue	Dead tissue.
Negative reinforcement	A behaviour that contributes to the removal of an aversive (painful) stimulus is likely to increase the probability of the occurrence of that particular behaviour.
Neonatal	Relates to newborn babies.
Nephritis	Inflammation of the kidney.
Neuralgia	Sharp, severe pain extending along a nerve or group of nerves.
Neuritis	Inflammation of the nerve.
Non-verbal communication	A form of communication that has body language as its foundation.
Obedience	Influence by order of authority.
Oedipus complex	This is a stage during child development where boys develop a special kind of affection for their mothers, whom they see as belonging to them and fathers are seen as rivals.
Operant conditioning	Behaviour is followed by a consequence, and the nature of the consequence influences an individual's tendency to repeat or not to repeat similar behaviour. For example, reward reinforces behaviour, whereas punishment will most likely eradicate it.
Overpersonal	The need to become extremely close to other people.
Oversocial	Also known as extrovert and would constantly seek other people's company because they can't bear to be on their own.
Palpitation	Irregular and rapid heartbeat.

Paralanguage	A mixture between verbal and non-verbal communication and includes silence, pause between words or sentences, tone, pitch, and speed of delivery.
Paranoid schizophrenia	A type of schizophrenia characterised by delusion of persecution and ideas of reference.
Paraphrasing	Restating the sentiments of what another person has said except in one's own words.
Patienthood	Assuming the role of patient.
Perceptual schemata	We each have our own way of looking at things.
Perinatal	Relates to the period around childbirth, in particular the five months before and one month after birth.
Personal helplessness	It is said to be present when people come to believe that they can't solve their problem but that the problem itself is not unsolvable.
Personal schema	The beliefs that we attribute to people, for example, we may see someone good or bad.
Personhood	Being a person with those qualities that confer distinct individuality.
Phenomenological world	An individual's subjective view of his or her world.
Phoneme	Basic unit of sound.
Pining	Hunger for desire or pangs of grief.
Pneumonia	Inflammation of the lungs.
Pneumothorax	Accumulation of air in the plural cavity of the lungs.
Political value	The need for power drives behaviour.
Polyuria	Excessive passage of urine as in diabetes.
Positive reinforcement	Reward reinforces behaviour.
Posture	Body language that reveals information within the context of a given situation and involves the whole of the body.
Power through	The capacity to affect others by influence and control.
Preconscious	Sometimes referred to as subconscious where information is not in our immediate awareness but can be easily recalled to consciousness.
Premorbid personality	The condition of a patient's personality before the onset of a disorder.
Prerequisite	Needed as a requirement.
Primary appraisal	Establishing the relevance and the impact of an event to oneself.

Problem-focused coping	Energy is spent by addressing the actual problem.
Prognosis	The outcome of an illness.
Projection	The unconscious rejection of emotional manifestation within oneself and attributing these onto others. For example, *I don't like you* becomes *you don't like me.*
Proxemics	The systematic study of these spatial features of social presentation or simply known as distance between interactants.
Proximity	Closeness.
Psychotic illness	A severe mental disorder, with or without organic damage, characterised by deterioration of personality and loss of contact with reality.
Punishment	A painful stimulus is inflicted in an attempt to prevent the repetition of the corresponding activity.
Rage	Violent and explosive anger.
Rationalisation	An unconscious process whereby a false but acceptable reason is given for behaviour that has in fact a much less acceptable motive.
Reaction formation	Adopting a behaviour opposite to that which reflects the individual's true feelings.
Real loss	Separation from the object of attachment has actually occurred.
Receptive aphasia	Also known as Wernicke's aphasia is the inability to understand the meaning of words.
Reflexivity	The turning back of one's experience on oneself.
Regression	Means stepping back to an earlier level of development.
Religious value	God has the answer to everything.
Repression	Unconscious turning of a traumatic event away from one's awareness.
Resistance stage	The body sets up its defence against the invading organisms.
Responsibility	Liability.
Role competence	The ability to recognise what is appropriate behaviour for a given role.
Role schemas	An expected set of behaviours from people depending on their role.
Rudimentary	Basic.
Schema	A hypothetical cognitive structure that people use to perceive, organise, process, and use information about the world.

Schizophrenia	One of the severe psychotic disorders characterised by distortions of reality, disturbances of thought and language, and withdrawal from social contact.
Secondary appraisal	Individuals evaluate whether or not they have sufficient resources to address the stressful stimulus.
Self	Those descriptions that we ascribe to ourselves.
Self-awareness	Self-knowledge or self-consciousness as in an ability to have insight into one's inner world and personality.
Self-centred bias	Also known as egocentric bias individuals take credit for more than their share of responsibility for a task that is performed by two or more people.
Self-competence	The ability to choose and portray a desired self-image. This means recognising one's strengths and weaknesses in a given situation.
Self-esteem	The value we hold of ourselves depending on our successes and failures.
Self-promotion	Tendency to show oneself as important by displaying one's certificates, awards, or posters in full view for everyone to see.
Self-schemas	An organised knowledge of self.
Self-serving bias	This is the tendency to attribute positive events to self and negative events to external factors.
Self-serving biases	Taking credit for success and denying responsibility for failure.
Self-transparent	Obvious to oneself.
Separation	To be apart.
Situational attribution	Also known as external attribution and where behaviour is linked to the situation. For example, I failed my exam because of the illegibility of the paper.
Sitz bath	A bathtub shaped like a chair in which one bathes in a sitting position, immersing only the hips and buttocks.
Social	People described as social feel comfortable with or without the company of other people.
Social cognition	The manner in which people interpret, analyse, and remember information about the social world.
Social feeling	Understanding the needs and goals of others during an interaction.
Social intelligence	To be socially intelligent means to possess the ability to get on with people in general as well as in social situation and knowing what to do in these situations.
Social judgement	The evaluation we make of people.

Social perception	The process whereby people form impressions of and make inferences about others.
Social value	People orientated.
Strain	This is seen as the outcome of stress, evidenced by some injury, the degree of which depends on the extent of the strain.
Stress	Feeling of being out of control in a given situation or in one's life.
Stressor	A stimulus that has the potential to lead to stress, seen as a negative response.
Succumbing	Giving way to.
Supplication	Giving the message that one is weak and that one needs help from others. Not dissimilar to playing the victim.
Suppression	The act of consciously pushing painful memories or negative experiences outside awareness.
Syntax	Arrangements of words that convey meaning.
Thanatos	Freudian concept for the instinct of death.
Theoretical values	Search for truth.
Thwarting	To upset or cause discomfort.
Transparency	Clearly visible.
TWOC	Taken With Out Consent.
Unconditional positive regard	Showing a warm, positive, and acceptant attitude towards another person free of conditions.
Underpersonal	The tendency to avoid close personal relationships with others and prefer to keep relationship at a superficial level.
Undersocial	Also known as introvert and would consciously establish and maintain distances between self and others.
Universal helplessness	Is said to be present when people come to believe a problem is unsolvable in that neither they nor anyone else can solve it.
Utilitarian or adaptive	Serving a purpose.
Values	Standards that we subscribe to in pursuit of our life goals.
Verbal communication	A form of communication that has speech and language as its foundation.
Vulnerability	In relation to stress, to be vulnerable means to be prone or susceptible to illness.
Yearning	Longing.

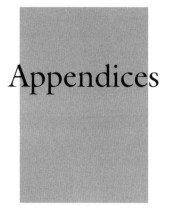

Appendices

Appendix I: Some of the words associated with 'power'

Force	Strength	Capacity	Ability	Control	Superior
Superior	Authority	Influence	Supremacy	Rule	Command
Clout	Muscle	Sway	Dominance	Vigour	Potency
Might	Energy	Greatness	Status	Calibre	Stamina
Paternalism	Choice	Independence	Decisions	Imposition	Instruct
Supervise	Manage	Oversee	Prescribe	Question	Challenge
Confront	Question	Dictate	Consult	Push	Punish
Knowledge	Steer	Predator	Manipulate	Boss	Cajole

Appendix 2: Some of the words associated with 'empowerment'

Give control	Informed choices	Independent	Participation	Influence	Gain mastery
Actively involved	Client focused	Autonomy	Equal partners	Options	Enhanced self-esteem
Sharing information	Power	Authorise	Permit	Approve	Endorse
Consent to	Knowledge	Validate	Esteem	Recognition	Respect
Enabling	Included as in social inclusion	Free to choose	Allowed to get it wrong	Questioning	Treat like an adult
Valuing difference	Individualised	Enhances self worth			

Appendix 3: Some of the words associated with 'loss'

Disable	Job	Illness	Terminal illness	Status	Control and power
Death	Trust	Hope	Independence	Limbs	Other body parts
Divorce	Physical	Continence	Cognitive functions	Missing	Home
Will to live	Suicide	Murder	Income	Friends	Sight (eyes)
Sound (hearing)	Self-esteem	Self-image	Theft and burglary	Confidence	Freedom
Accidents	Sexual function	Inability to conceive	Deprivation	Safety	Security
Virginity					

Appendix 4: Possible hindrances for reinvesting energy into another relationship

Fear that future relationship may end in a similar way	What will the children say?	Not fair on the children	Married for life	Can't love another person the same way	Feel they are betraying the dead person
Promise never to love again					

Appendix 5: Factors that could hinder the grieving process

Unresolved issues in relationship (I wish I could have told him or her in the living years)	Unresolved issues in relationship (I wish I could have told him or her in the living years)	Been together for a long time	Unexpected and sudden death	Anger	Only just started your relationship: not enough time
Vulnerability, for example, personality	Vulnerability, for example, personality	What the loss means	Perceived responsibility as in 'it's my fault'	Guilt and blame	Lack of support
Non-disclosing (don't want to talk about it)	Non-disclosing (don't want to talk about it)	Nature of death, for example, Tsunamis, murders, body never found	Multiple losses (the loss of more than one person in a family)	Loss that is not talked about, for example, rape, abuse	Taboo subject, for example, HIV and AIDS, suicide, suicide bombers and criminals
Distance, for example, someone dies far away from you					

Appendix 6: Some forms of aggression

Failing to warn someone of the impending danger	Talking about others behind their backs	Failing to pass on important information to others	Failing to defend others. Belittling others	Giving the silent treatment. Rude gestures	Constantly interrupting. Ridiculing others
Leaving on purpose when the target person enters the room	Condescending	Failing to deny rumours. Sexual remarks	Deliberatly being late for meeting	Sabotage. Withholding information	Physical attack
Verbal abuse	Thieving	Threatening physical violence	Destroying mails addressed to others	Damaging property. Staring	Self-harming behaviour
Sulking	Suicide and homicide	Force feeding	Being sarcastic	Bullying	Being ironic
Jealousy	Envy	Loss of self-control	Invasion of personal space		

Author Index

Subject Index

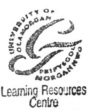